MANAGING
HERPES

MANAGING HERPES

LIVING & LOVING
WITH HSV

BY CHARLES EBEL &
ANNA WALD, M.D., M.P.H.

AMERICAN SOCIAL HEALTH ASSOCIATION

RESEARCH TRIANGLE PARK, NORTH CAROLINA

AMERICAN SOCIAL HEALTH ASSOCIATION, INC.
P. O. Box 13827
Research Triangle Park, North Carolina 27709
www.ASHAstd.org

Book Design: Cate Rogers
Layout: Cate Rogers
Illustrations: pp. 11, 35, 40, 41, 42, 43—Mike Dulude

Library of Congress Control Number: 2007929553
ISBN-13: 978-1-885833-08-2

Printed in the United States of America.

DEDICATION

In memory of Stephen Sacks, M.D., and Stephen Straus, M.D., who brought warmth, wisdom, and scientific excellence to this field of research.

CONTENTS

CONTENTS

CONTENTS

PREFACE

A book such as this always forces the writer to ask what has changed-in this case over the five years since our 2002 edition. The answer, at first, seemed to be very little. But as we worked through the 19 chapters we found many topics that required significant updates.

While there has not been a spectacular research breakthrough to redefine medical management or dramatically change perceptions, there are encouraging developments for people with herpes. Perhaps most importantly, research has confirmed the role of an oral antiviral drug in reducing the risk of transmitting herpes to a sexual partner, and we now have several studies showing that condoms protect against transmitting or getting herpes as well.

We have also seen major gains in the area of herpes diagnostics. The type-specific blood tests we wrote about in 2002, still relatively new and not widely adopted by clinical practitioners, are now offered by major commercial laboratories and available to a great many more people. This development, along with the today's larger number of dosing schedules for antiviral drugs, suggest an overall improvement in the quality of care for herpes. Unlike the era of the 1990s in which our first edition was first published, relatively few patients today will be told they "just have to live with it."

While we are still on hold for a Nobel-prize caliber blockbuster, the research pipeline is intriguing. Interest in new vaccine approaches is still high, and the recognized role of herpes simplex as a cofactor in worldwide HIV/AIDS epidemic may help to attract funding to the vaccine area.

In short, patients have more resources for managing herpes today than they did just five short years ago.

Charles Ebel
Anna Wald, M.D., M.P.H.

ACKNOWLEDGMENTS

As *Managing Herpes* evolves yet again with this new publication in 2007, it remains appropriate to acknowledge several past and present members of ASHA's Scientific Advisory Committee on herpes who contributed greatly to the educational work that shaped this content. They include Lawrence Corey, M.D., Stephen Straus, M.D., Gray Davis, Ph.D., Zane Brown, M.D., Sevgi Aral, Ph D, Edward Hook, III, M.D., Lawrence Stanberry, M.D., Ph.D., Susan Rosenthal, PhD, and Joan Wiebel, R.N.C.

It is also fitting to acknowledge ASHA staff and consultants who have played a role in creating new educational content on HSV over the past few years, especially Lisa Hyatt Smith, Rachele Peterson, Joanne Grosshans, and Fred Wyand. Thanks as well to Lynn Barclay for all the "cat-herding" necessary to bring the book to print and to Cate Rogers for typesetting and cover design.

I'm indebted to Rhoda Ashley, PhD, and Zane Brown, MD, for reviewing portions of this text. And to the staff of the Virology Research Clinic at the University of Washington for all their hospitality during a "writing vacation" in February 2007.

1

THE NEWS

"I had been managing on my own as a single parent for nine years," says Carolyn, "and I'd decided to pursue what I thought might be a promising relationship with a man I'd recently met. Several weeks later, there I was at the gynecologist's office, hearing that I might have genital herpes. The doctor gave me some printed material and a prescription, and told me she would have lab results in about a week. At the pharmacy next door I was holding back tears, wanting to hide from everyone, somehow feeling they were all staring at me. When I got to my car, I drove straight home and read the material over and over, hoping to find I had something else."

For some, a diagnosis of genital herpes comes as a complete shock. They know next to nothing about herpes, and they perceive themselves to be at zero risk of sexually transmitted infections (STIs). For others, it's not as big a surprise. They may have had a partner who had it or may know enough about its symptoms to make an educated guess. Many first learn they have herpes when they seek medical attention for some kind of symptom in the genital area, though they might not have suspected that herpes would be the explanation. For a few, a herpes diagnosis is the result of a blood test taken as part of a broader work-up for sexually transmitted infections.

Whatever the circumstances, it's safe to say nobody *likes* getting diagnosed with genital herpes. Some may see it as a relatively minor issue—the inevitable price of being sexually active—yet still not good news. For others, it's a traumatic event, capable of causing a range of emotions.

One of the factors that gives herpes the potential to cause distress is the fact that it's a sexually transmitted infection. Growing up in American society, many of us come to view an STI like gonorrhea or syphilis—or, more recently, herpes—as something strange and horrible that happens only to those who have done something wrong. People who deserve trouble in their lives. People of bad morals. Attitudes about STIs vary depending on religion and a number of other cultural factors, but many of us have a hard time accepting the fact that we have an infection spread through having sex. It's often something about which we're taught to feel ashamed—or at least embarrassed.

Is this a reasonable attitude? Certainly few people would go out of their way to acquire an STI. Most of us would prefer to remain free of illnesses, whatever they might be. But the fact remains that all of us get sick during our lives. All of us are exposed to, and ultimately infected with, a host of bacteria and viruses that pose challenges to our health. Some of these germs are spread through the air or food or through contact with household objects that have been in some way contaminated. Some are spread through close physical contact with another person, including sexual contact.

Most of us are astonished to learn that infections spread through *sexual contact* are among the most widespread in our society. In fact, among infectious diseases only the common cold surpasses STIs in the number of people affected. According to the latest figures from the U.S. Centers for Disease Control and Prevention (CDC), there are more than 19 million new cases of sexually transmitted infections every year. *That's 52,054 people, newly infected, every day—enough to fill Franklin Field in Philadelphia.*

When you think about it, the fact that STIs are so rampant shouldn't come as such a huge surprise. After all, people in all walks of life do have sex. It's as much a part of our biological make-up as eating and sleeping. And when we have sex, we sometimes pass a variety of common germs back and forth. One of the most common, it turns out, is herpes simplex virus (HSV), the cause of genital herpes. This particular infection is a fact of life for roughly 50 million people in the U.S.—something on the order of one in five persons over the age of 14. An increasing number of us understand how prevalent herpes is, but most, ironically, do not translate this information into a sense of personal risk. Despite what we know "on paper," we tend to see herpes as something that will happen only to someone else.

It's normal to feel some embarrassment about getting any sexually transmitted infection, even to feel that this condition somehow separates you from your friends, or changes the way you will interact with them. But getting an STI is hardly a rare event. And as you can see, getting herpes puts you in rather large company.

All this is not to say that you don't have a right to your feelings If a herpes diagnosis has caused you distress. Herpes is for all of us an unwelcome guest, and one of the things about it that is so distressing is that it's probably a lifelong guest. Often the first questions we ask the doctor in that fateful office visit focus on getting rid of it. "What do we do about it? What drug can I take? What's the cure?"

The answer, as you probably know by now, is that medical science as yet has no cure for herpes. There are a number of medications that can help to control herpes, although none can wipe it out entirely. Some people choose to rely on these to keep herpes under control, while others come to feel that they don't need any medicines. Researchers, of course, are still hard at work, and the search for new drugs continues. Several types of vaccines are also in development.

In the meantime, it's important to remember that, *with time,* most people find herpes is not the catastrophe it might seem to be at the start. The physical and emotional distress of herpes usually peaks early on, often in the first few months.

The experience of millions of people shows that herpes does not have to be—and usually isn't—a major, life-changing event. Depending on the circumstances, and the type of symptoms involved, it often does require a process of adjustment—in our view of ourselves, in our relationships, and sometimes in the way we approach our physical health and well-being. The first step is to gain a better understanding about herpes and the issues it might raise in our lives.

By opening this book, you've already taken that first step.

2

A VIRUS
IS A VIRUS
IS A VIRUS?

Herpes is caused by a virus—herpes simplex virus (HSV). In order to understand herpes more fully, it's important to start with the big picture and go over some key facts about viral infection in general. This chapter doesn't deal directly with many of the practical issues you may be facing if you're just recently diagnosed with herpes, but stay with it: A grounding in some of the basics here may help you later as you try to answer some of your own specific questions about genital herpes.

You may or may not remember much about viruses from high school biology, but you've been coping with them for most of your life. There are dozens of families of viruses and hundreds of individual types. Rhinoviruses, for example, are the frequent culprit in the common cold. Influenza viruses cause the respiratory ailment known as the flu. And a host of enteroviruses cause the intestinal disorders that almost everyone copes with from time to time. Other infectious diseases caused by viruses run the gamut from measles to hepatitis to HIV.

HERPESVIRUSES: THE FAMILY TREE

Some people find the term *herpesvirus* confusing. Spelled out as one word, *herpesvirus* actually refers to a family of viruses with certain traits in common. This family includes Epstein-Barr virus, the cause of infectious mononucleosis ("mono"); varicella zoster, the cause of chickenpox in children and shingles in adults; and herpes simplex, the cause of cold sores on the face as well as genital herpes. (See table below.) The recently discovered herpesviruses—HHV-6, HHV-7, and HHV-8—may cause illness in some people who have normal immune systems but are more likely to cause health problems in those who have suppressed immune function. Research on these relatively new viruses remains in its early stages.

HUMAN HERPESVIRUSES

HERPES SIMPLEX VIRUS, TYPE 1	HSV-1
HERPES SIMPLEX VIRUS, TYPE 2	HSV-2
EPSTEIN-BARR VIRUS	EBV
VARICELLA ZOSTER VIRUS	VZV
CYTOMEGALOVIRUS	CMV
HUMAN HERPESVIRUSES, TYPE 6	HHV-6
HUMAN HERPESVIRUSES, TYPE 7	HHV-7
HUMAN HERPESVIRUSES, TYPE 8	HHV-8

As you can see from this family tree, most of us have had dealings with at least a couple of herpesviruses by the time we reach adulthood. Almost all of us, for example, are infected with varicella zoster as children. We suffer through the usual drudgery of chickenpox—the fever, the sores—until we pull through and shake the infection. Similarly, many of us have experienced a bout with "mono" sometime in our teens or early twenties.

Like all other viruses, a herpesvirus makes its way in the world by living in healthy cells. Once it gets a hold in the body, it finds a way to invade normal cells and disrupt their usual functions. The virus uses the machinery of the normal cell to produce more copies of itself, a process called *viral replication.*

Many viral infections defy treatment—they can't be cured the way antibiotics cure strep throat. Though gains have been made recently in treating influenza and several other viruses, scientists generally have found it difficult to stop viral infections. The classic example is the common cold or the intestinal virus that takes us to the family doctor looking for relief. The usual response goes something like, "It's probably just a virus—there's not much we can do except to let it run its course."

In reality, a virus doesn't simply "run its course," tiring out and quitting by itself. Rather, it's our set of natural defenses—the immune system—that finally halts the illness brought on by viral invaders. The process may take days or weeks, but with the most common viruses the immune system eventually wins out, and the virus is eliminated. End of story.

Unfortunately, with herpesviruses the story has another chapter. The catch is that the herpesviruses find a way to retreat from the immune system and persist in the body without causing any symptoms. This ability to persist—to find a permanent hideaway—is called *latency.* Once established, latent herpesvirus infections are capable of remaining in a dormant phase, sometimes for long periods of time. Latent herpes infections, however, also are capable of becoming active again at unpredictable times. When this happens, the virus begins to replicate and sometimes causes symptoms of illness similar to those it brought on the first time. The majority of the herpes-viruses—including HSV-1 and HSV-2—follow this pattern.

The most familiar example of this cycle of initial infection, latency, and reactivation is probably that of varicella zoster, which causes chickenpox. As children, almost all of us are exposed to varicella zoster and thus develop a case of those annoying little sores all over the body, along with fever and other symptoms of infection. In time, the sores heal and we recover. What's more, our bodies have perfected the strategy for an immune system attack on varicella zoster. So the next time we're exposed, we don't get sick—we have developed an *immunity*. It is nonetheless possible to have a flare-up of herpes zoster later in life, which is called *shingles*. This second episode is brought on by the virus that has been hiding away in the nerve roots inside our own bodies—not by exposure to someone else who is sick. This is a simple illustration of latency and reactivation.

HERPES SIMPLEX VIRUS (HSV)

With this as background, let's look more closely at HSV and how it's going to affect you and your health.

To begin with, there are two distinct types of HSV. These look almost identical under a microscope and have many of the same properties. The chief difference between them is that they have marked preferences when it comes to where they live. HSV-1 prefers to live above the waist. It's best known as the cause of the fever blisters or cold sores that people get around the lips, mouth, and nose. HSV-2 prefers to live below the waist. There it can produce sores on the genitals that sometimes resemble cold sores.

While the two types of HSV have *sites of preference,* as researchers call them, they are also somewhat adaptable. HSV-1 is capable of gaining a hold and causing trouble in the genital area. Likewise, HSV-2 can occasionally bring about cold sores on the face. More on this later.

How It Spreads

HSV spreads from person to person through direct contact. Unlike common cold viruses that may pass through the air when someone sneezes, and unlike an enterovirus that might find its way to you on a contaminated piece of food, HSV generally requires skin-to-skin contact as a route of travel. It also requires a target area of skin that is vulnerable to its advances. Some types of skin cells— the soft skin of the genitals, for example, or the moist surfaces of mucous membranes such as in the mouth, vagina, and anus—offer relatively easy access for the invading HSV. The thicker skin of the arms, torso, and legs, by contrast, provides a barrier to HSV. At these sites, HSV can take hold only if the skin is damaged. This concept will be discussed further in later chapters.

With these facts in mind, consider three very basic scenarios:

• A person with a cold sore caused by HSV-1 kisses someone on the mouth and spreads the virus. This causes the second person to get cold sores on the mouth as well.

• A person with genital herpes caused by HSV-2 has sexual intercourse with a partner and spreads the virus, causing the partner to develop genital herpes.

• A person with HSV-1 cold sores performs oral sex on a partner, causing the partner to develop genital herpes sores. In this scenario, we have genital herpes caused by HSV-1.

The spread of herpes is a complicated subject, and it's discussed in more detail later. For now, the important point to remember is that HSV spreads through skin-to-skin contact, from an area of skin where virus is present to a skin site that is susceptible.

Active and Inactive Phases: A Thumbnail "History"

What happens when HSV gets in your body? Once infected, the pattern and timing of events differ somewhat from person to person, but the basics remain the same. Once HSV gains a foothold, the virus begins replicating, spreading, and invading the local nerve cells. As we mentioned earlier, the defining event of infection is latency—the virus' successful effort to set up a permanent base of operations. With HSV, this process of latency occurs in the nerve roots. Having traveled the nerve pathways, HSV finds safe sanctuary in nests of nerve cells termed *sensory ganglia*. These lie near, but outside of, the spinal cord and the bony vertebral column. In cases of genital herpes, HSV retreats to the sacral ganglia, located near the base of the spine (see Figure 1). In oral-facial herpes, HSV finds its way to the trigeminal ganglia, near the top of the spine. In these ganglia, the virus remains safe from the immune system and is capable of returning to an active state, though it can remain inactive for various periods of time.

The appearance of signs and symptoms during HSV's initial invasion is a tricky issue. The process of infection and latency requires only a few days. Therefore, the virus has become entrenched *before* a person might experience symptoms. Many people who develop symptoms will notice them within the first 10 days. On the other hand, one's first encounter with HSV may cause changes so subtle

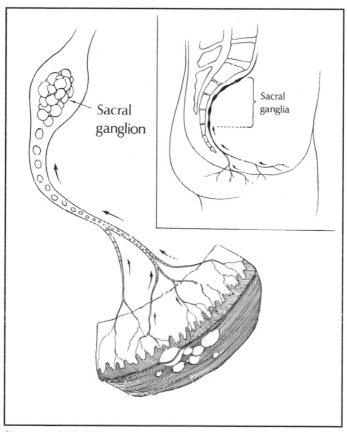

FIGURE 1. *HSV retreats along the nerves and finds sanctuary in the sacral ganglia, shown here.*

that they aren't recognized. We'll discuss this in more detail in the next few chapters.

Beyond the initial infection and establishment of latency, there is also the prospect of reactivation. When HSV is latent, various biological events can cause it to become active and begin traveling the nerve pathways from the ganglia back to the skin. There it can cause signs and symptoms once more (or perhaps for the first time).

How Common Is It?

Some people are shocked to learn how widespread herpes simplex is. Researchers estimate that 58% of all Americans between the ages of 14 and 49 are infected with HSV-1, most of which represents cold sores—oral herpes. Some people get an initial HSV-1 infection and have a bout with cold sores in childhood and then have no recurrences of the infection in their adult lives. Studies show that only about a third of those with latent HSV-1 report having had flare-ups with visible cold sores. HSV-1, then, is for the most part a commonplace and very benign infection. Only about 1 in 10 infected persons, or approximately 15 million, will experience recurrent oral-facial herpes several times per year.

HSV-2 is not as widespread, but it's hardly a rarity. The most authoritative national survey, the National Health and Nutrition Examination Study (NHANES), published new data on HSV-2 in late 2006. Researchers analyzing this data report that 20% of Americans between the ages of 20 and 49 have HSV-2 infection. While the rates of HSV-2 are much less than this among teens, and higher among persons over the age of 50, we can say as an average that HSV-2 is present in one in five adults, which equates to approximately 50 million people. Interestingly, the previous published figures, based on NHANES data from the early 1990s, estimated HSV-2 prevalence to be somewhat higher. In the interim there appears to have been a decline in new infection rates among people in their teens and early twenties. At the same time, the number of people with genital herpes caused by HSV-1 has increased. For one thing, people are more susceptible to HSV-1 nowadays than they were just a few decades ago. It's also possible there is an increase of oral sex among adolescents who are initiating sexual activity, as an alternative to vaginal sex.

If you're having trouble believing there are so many people with genital herpes, bear in mind that most don't know they have it. Researchers can test blood samples in a population to find out what percentage have HSV-2. When they interview those who test positive, *about 85% say they have never had herpes symptoms!* In studies where these apparently symptom-free individuals are questioned further, a majority will recall some minor genital symptoms that they had never thought of as herpes. The other group holds to its initial testimony: No history of genital sores or the like.

What makes one person react so differently from another when infected with the same virus? Some scientists guess that these differences reflect variations in the individuals' immune responses; others suspect they center on the actual quantity of virus one is infected with, or on the particular strain of the virus involved. As yet, however, researchers can't fully explain the huge variability in herpes symptoms among equally healthy adults.

THE BOTTOM LINE

To cut through all the science, keep in mind a couple of very basic facts:

First, if you have HSV, you have in your body a virus that operates, in most ways, just like dozens of other viruses you've carried around from time to time. The trouble with herpes simplex is that your immune system can't completely get rid of it. The virus can hide away and enjoy a lengthy stay through latency.

Second, you're not alone. The majority of adults carry around some form of herpes simplex, either type 1 or type 2—or both. They may not know it, because it may cause mild symptoms or no symptoms at all. Either way, however, with a latent infection like herpes simplex, the potential for viral reactivation persists.

So, medically speaking, herpes is neither an exotic nor an especially dangerous infection in the vast majority of people. We're talking about a "garden variety" bug. No more, no less.

3

THE STI YOU DIDN'T KNOW YOU HAD?

THE STI YOU DIDN'T KNOW YOU HAD?

"My partner and I didn't want to be taking any risks in this new relationship," says Shelley, "so we decided we'd get HIV tests and get checked for other STIs. At my clinic, when I asked about STI tests, they told me there's a new blood test for herpes and asked if I wanted that included in my STI screening. I said yes. Well, the result was positive for HSV-2. I was stunned. At first, I thought it had to be a mistake. 'I've never had this,' I told them. Never had anything wrong sexually. But now that I've read more about it, I can see that herpes can be a sort of silent thing. Anyway, what I'm wondering is: What now? Do I need to do something about it?"

Many readers of this book probably have had symptoms of genital herpes, and the way they view it is colored by the physical reality of it. As new technologies take hold, however, it's likely that a significant number of readers are being diagnosed based on type-specific blood tests—tests that work in the absence of symptoms.

The most extensive study to date on the prevalence of genital herpes is called the National Health and Nutrition Examination Survey (NHANES). The method in this NHANES survey is to collect blood and other samples from thousands of persons who represent a cross-section of the U.S. population, and test these samples for a variety of medical conditions. One of these tests identifies the presence of herpes simplex virus type 2 (HSV-2). The 2006 results showed that 17% of the U.S. population between the ages of 14 and 49 had HSV-2 infection. Even more surprising than this, however, was the percentage of those who are apparently symptom-free. When interviewed about a past history of genital herpes symptoms, a full 85% of those infected with HSV-2 gave no history of symptoms.

As you can see from the Figure 2, the proportion of genital herpes cases in which there are symptoms that cause someone to seek medical care is quite small. But there is more to the story.

A number of smaller studies using these specialized blood tests have made similar findings: That is, 80% to 90% of persons who have HSV-2 infection report no history of symptoms. In some of these

History vs. No History

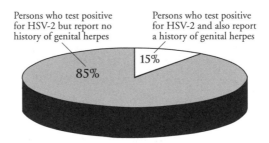

FIGURE 2. *The NHANES survey shows that only 15% of those testing positive for HSV-2 are aware that they have genital herpes.*

smaller studies, however, researchers were able to develop a more in-depth profile of these apparently asymptomatic individuals and understand what was behind the statistics. For example, they spent time teaching the study recruits about herpes, and in particular used photographs to show examples of the types of signs and symptoms than can be associated with genital herpes—some of which are quite subtle. This educational process yielded another surprising result: After a few months, up to 62% of those who initially reported no history of symptoms were reporting that they could now recognize some form of herpes. Figure 3 on this page shows an overlay of this data on the NHANES data. It suggests that while only 15% of those with HSV-2 have obvious recognized symptoms, perhaps as many as 70% have unrecognized symptoms. In many cases these individuals had sought care for genital symptoms but had indeterminate test results or were incorrectly diagnosed with another condition.

Unrecognized vs. Asymptomatic Infection

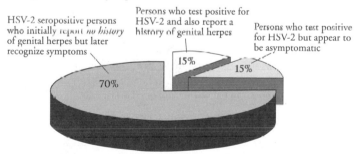

FIGURE 3. *This figure illustrates the phenomenon of unrecognized herpes: While 85% of those testing positive for HSV-2 initially give no history of herpes, the majority of this group is likely to recognize herpes symptoms when educated.*

In any case, before we delve into more details describing symptoms, treatments, and how the virus behaves over a long period of time, it makes sense to address the question: *What sort of herpes information is relevant to the person who hasn't had any signs or symptoms— or at least, not any he or she is aware of?*

In general, most of the scientific research on herpes over the past half-century has been conducted on people who do have symptoms. However, since the mid-1980s, as scientists perfected HSV blood tests, we are beginning to learn much more about the large number of people who either have no symptoms or who have subtle, unrecognized symptoms. The findings of this research suggest that on some counts HSV operates the same way in persons with mild or unrecognized symptoms as it does in persons with obvious recurrent infections:

• All persons who are antibody-positive for HSV have latent infections, as described in the last chapter. HSV has established a permanent base of operations in the nerve ganglia. For HSV-2 (genital herpes), this is most likely to be the sacral nerve ganglia.

• Most people who test positive for HSV-2 and never recall having symptoms actually do have very mild symptoms they can learn to recognize as herpes.

• Whether a person experiences obvious symptoms or not, HSV-2 does reactivate from time to time, traveling the nerve pathways. Thus, there are times a person with unrecognized herpes might transmit herpes to a sexual partner.

There are, of course, other differences as well. Readers who have been diagnosed solely on the basis of a blood test may find the description of *first episodes* to be completely unfamiliar. Likewise, the observations here on patterns of recurrences over the long term may not apply. Those who have never had herpes symptoms may also take a very different view on the need for—or role of—treatment.

Equally important, our description of the emotional and psychosocial issues associated with herpes might also ring false. If you feel that this book overstates the psychological impact of a herpes diagnosis, that is perhaps because the existing literature on herpes is drawn mostly from those with symptomatic recurrences. As we suggest in Chapter 1, in our limited experience with serologic testing thus far, a positive result for HSV-2 is seldom welcome news, but most people adjust well fairly quickly. In several studies, those diagnosed in this way did experience some initial distress as indicated by standardized instruments for measuring changes in mood, but over time there were no significant changes in life quality, sexual satisfaction, or optimism.

As we have constructed this edition of *Managing Herpes,* we have attempted to keep in mind the fact that readers may have broadly diverse experiences with genital herpes. All the same, if you have been diagnosed based on a blood test, like Shelley in the beginning of this chapter, you may find yourself wanting to skip over some of the material. However, we suggest that you pay special attention to a number of specific chapters:

Chapter 5, "Recurrent Genital Herpes: The Long Run"— Because so many people can learn to recognize subtle signs and symptoms of herpes recurrences, the description of symptoms in this chapter may be helpful. In addition, there is information here about HSV's cycle of dormant and active phases.

Chapter 6, "How Is Herpes Spread?" and Chapter 7, "Who's To Blame?"—These chapters address the confusion that people might have about how they have acquired herpes and concerns about when and how they can transmit herpes to sexual partners.

Chapter 8, "Patient and Provider" and Chapter 9, "Treatment Options"— If you have never yet had symptoms, you may see little purpose in seeing a medical professional about herpes, but the time may come when you do need treatment or professional consultation. The first of these two chapters outlines some of the benefits of getting professional care and offers suggestions on how to approach the issue with your provider. The second explores current FDA-approved treatment options.

Chapter 11, "Sorting Out the Emotional Issues"— If getting a positive test result has been traumatic, this chapter may be a useful tool in thinking through the next steps.

Chapter 13, "Herpes and Your Sex Life"— A high percentage of people who have genital herpes are concerned about the effect it will have on their sexual relationships—and especially about the risk of transmission. This chapter explains the risk of transmission in couples and explores options for reducing that risk.

Chapter 14, "Herpes and Pregnancy"— The risks of transmitting herpes to a newborn—though a rare event—should be understood by every couple in which one or both partners have herpes. Men, too, should be educated on this topic, because the highest risk of neonatal herpes arises in couples in which the expectant mother acquires herpes *during* pregnancy.

IN THE END, the person who as yet has had no symptoms may have an easier time managing herpes as a health issue. But there are still several key aspects of this viral infection that will be worth your while to understand well.

MANAGING HERPES

4

THE FIRST EPISODE: HSV'S INITIAL IMPACT

"I was shell-shocked over having herpes anyway," says Erik. "But I was also pretty sick. I had wet blisters on my genitals, I itched like I had poison ivy, and I felt really run-down, too. It was almost like mono, with a sore throat and swollen glands. I don't know whether I was depressed or just sick, but I also felt listless—didn't want to do anything. I just lay in bed most of the time, and missed a couple of days of work. When the medication kicked in, I could see the sores healing up and I started to feel better. But it was two weeks before all the symptoms were gone."

As we mentioned in the previous chapter, many people infected with herpes simplex virus (HSV) either have no symptoms or, more likely, mild symptoms that they don't recognize as herpes. But a significant number will have symptoms of the infection right from the beginning. For many, like Erik, the trouble begins with a very difficult period of illness called a first episode. This is likely to last longer and to cause more discomfort and stress than symptomatic periods that might occur later.

THE IMMUNE RESPONSE

First episodes are capable of stirring up considerable trouble because the invading virus has the element of surprise. Your body's defenses are not prepared for herpes. It takes a while before the immune system can identify the invader and refine its weapons to combat HSV. As it does, your immune response will succeed first in slowing the invasion and finally in forcing HSV to retreat from the field of battle.

Unfortunately, this doesn't happen overnight. The body's natural defense needs careful coordination among various parts of the immune system. These include the cellular immune response (the work of lymphocytes and macrophages) and the humoral immune response (antibodies). Using a combination of defenses, your body will try to kill the virus as it moves from cell to cell, get rid of cells already infected, and try to protect cells that are still healthy.

As all this microscopic warfare is carried out, it may take several weeks before any progress can be made against the invading virus. But in the long run there is good news. After its initial struggle with HSV, your immune system will remain prepared for future encounters. For example, the body keeps on making the specific antibodies that cripple the virus, and they will work more quickly the next time HSV emerges from the nerve roots.

How long a first episode lasts will vary a great deal from person to person. Probably the most important factor is your prior history with HSV.

Let's say that you've never had either HSV-1 or HSV-2 before. Through sexual contact you become infected with genital herpes caused by HSV-2. This is not only your first encounter with HSV-2, it's your body's first glimpse at herpes simplex of either type. So the virus is able to replicate and spread before the body can mount an effective counterattack. The same scenario might occur with a first exposure to HSV-1 as well. In either case, because your immune system has no direct experience with HSV, the body takes time to marshal its forces, and the signs and symptoms of infection can be severe.

By contrast, let's say that you're one of the many people who was exposed to HSV-1 as a child and has had the virus for years, whether you know it or not. At age 25, you become infected with HSV-2 through sexual contact and develop symptoms. Your immune system has seen HSV-1 before, but HSV-2 is a slightly different entity. Your natural defenses react much more quickly than in the first example, but they aren't able to keep herpes in check. Here, too, signs and symptoms often follow, though they're often not as dramatic as those in the first example.

In the scientific literature, these two kinds of first episodes are sometimes given different names. The first kind, in which a person has never had either type of HSV before, is often called a *primary first episode* or *true primary*. The second type, in which the person infected with HSV-2 is already infected with HSV-1, is called a *nonprimary first episode*. In this book, however, we will simply use the term first episode to describe any early symptoms resulting from initial infection with HSV of either type.

FIRST-EPISODE SYMPTOMS

If the process of infection is going to produce marked symptoms, these symptoms typically start within the first 10 days after exposure to HSV. Often the first sign of trouble is genital itching or pain, followed by a red spot or some other change in the skin on or near the genitals. Next comes the emergence of sores or *lesions*. (The scientific literature uses the term *lesion* to describe a wide range of abnormalities in body tissue, such as any break or irregularity in the skin.)

In first-episode genital herpes, lesions may appear in men on the penis and urethra, the scrotum, the upper thigh, or around the anus. In women, they are commonly found on the vulva (lips of the vagina), urethra, cervix, the upper thigh, or around the anus. The illustrations on pages 40-43 show these locations.

When initially seeing a healthcare provider, people with first-episode genital herpes usually have several lesions in different places in the genital area. About half the time, these are followed by a new crop of lesions in the second week. All in all, first-episode lesions will cause pain or discomfort for an average of 9-12 days and will take two to three weeks to heal fully. Lastly, as in the case of Erik, up to one-half of patients with first episodes experience more generalized symptoms, such as fever, malaise, headaches, and swollen glands, especially the lymph nodes near the groin. These generalized or "systemic" symptoms are more common in women than men.

First-episode lesions often follow a predictable sequence. Classic herpes skin lesions develop into fluid-filled vesicles that eventually form a crust and then a scab before healing completely. Lesions on mucosal tissue are typically ulcers that heal without scabbing. Residual scarring of any kind is rare in either type of location.

In addition to these "classic" symptoms, however, genital HSV infection can show itself in numerous ways. Lesions may be almost invisible to the naked eye or may look like a small pimple or insect bite, perhaps going unnoticed. Because of their varied appearance, herpes symptoms sometimes are mistaken for heat rash, jock itch, or ingrown hairs. Sometimes lesions will be extremely painful to the touch; sometimes they will not. The wide range of symptoms and their similarity to other conditions is one of the major reasons why so many of those who have genital herpes don't know it. (See Chapter 5 for more detail on the conditions that can be confused with genital herpes.)

When a first episode produces classic herpes lesions, healthcare providers often diagnose the condition based on the appearance of the lesions and the flu-like symptoms that frequently go along with them. First episodes can also lead to a number of other complications. One is difficulty in urinating. Lesions in or around the urethra itself can make it painful to pass urine, a problem that is more common in women with first episodes. If you have this problem, experts recommend that you urinate in a warm bath to ease the pain of contact with undiluted urine. In a small number of cases, the infection might actually affect the nerves that control urination, causing the patient to start retaining urine, a more serious problem requiring special medical care.

Some patients with a first episode also experience *aseptic meningitis.* This sounds serious but usually denotes only an intense headache. Meningitis brings with it a stiff neck and sometimes extra sensitivity to light or loud noises. For reasons unknown, this too is particularly common in women. In the end, meningitis that results from HSV resolves by itself and rarely recurs.

Though technically not a symptom, another potential problem with first episodes is the risk of spreading herpes to another part of the body. With first episodes there is more virus on the skin, and it persists for longer periods of time. Because the immune system hasn't yet set up a solid defense for herpes simplex, it's possible to spread HSV from one part of your body to another part during this period—a phenomenon called *autoinoculation.* This sometimes happens when a person touches a herpes sore and then quickly touches another part of the body, which can have the effect of transporting a small colony of virus to a new site where it has the chance to replicate and spread. One example of this would be the person who touches a genital herpes sore with a finger that has been abraded or cut recently. A herpes sore on the finger might result.

Studies suggest that autoinoculation occurs in only a small percentage of people with a primary first episode and is less common with other first episodes. After the immune response to herpes is fully established, autoinoculation is no longer an issue.

Lastly, the classic herpes lesions of a first episode may be susceptible to *superinfection.* In other words, the herpes lesions might become infected with fungus or bacteria, just as a cut in the skin might become infected. In women this may take the form of a vaginal yeast infection.

THE EMOTIONAL SIDE

The long list of symptoms is important to people with a first episode of genital herpes, but physical discomfort is only one piece of the problem. The American Social Health Association (ASHA) has heard from hundreds of thousands of herpes patients over the years, and the weight of evidence from these contacts suggests that the first episode of genital herpes also brings on the most intense emotions. Behavioral research and in-depth surveys also suggest an emotional impact that peaks in the first few months after a herpes diagnosis.

In a 1991 survey, for example, ASHA found that more than half of the 3,000 respondents noted feelings of depression, isolation, and fear of rejection during their initial outbreak. At the center of these feelings, people worried about the potential impact of herpes on their most intimate relationships. They experienced fears about the ways that herpes might change their sex lives. Some began to feel differently about themselves. Of equal importance, however, the survey also showed that these concerns diminish over time for a great number of people. The potential distress caused by herpes, including its sexual impact, will be discussed more fully in Chapters 11, 12, and 13.

WHAT YOU CAN DO

If you're experiencing your first bout with genital herpes, you're facing a host of issues and important personal decisions, such as whom to tell and how. Many of these questions are explored in detail in later chapters. The most immediate issues, meanwhile, are probably medical. Here is a brief list of steps that may help to keep the pain and anxiety of a first episode to a minimum:

• If you haven't already seen a doctor or other qualified health care professional, do this right away. With symptoms such as fever, headache, and swollen glands, you have every reason to seek a professional consultation. In particular, find out for sure whether you do indeed have herpes. For this, you often need a laboratory test, since there are other infections that can cause symptoms similar to first-episode HSV. Some patients try to diagnose themselves and later regret it, always wondering if it's really herpes.

• A number of diagnostic tests are available (see Chapter 16), some more accurate than others. Find out which test your healthcare provider uses and find out whether your symptoms are caused by HSV-1 or HSV-2. In the long run you will need this information to make decisions about your health.

• Discuss treatment options (Chapters 9 and 10). Antiviral drugs such as acyclovir or related compounds, such as famciclovir or valacyclovir, can hasten the healing process in first episodes, sometimes by several days. Treatment also dramatically reduces the duration of systemic complications, including meningitis. If you are facing pain and discomfort, the most decisive step you can take is antiviral treatment.

• For added help with troublesome lesions, consider taking a quick warm bath a couple of times a day. Some people say these provide excellent temporary relief. After the bath, be careful to dry the infected area gently with a soft towel, or use a hair dryer on the low setting. Keeping the area clean and dry relieves discomfort and can speed healing. The use of topical creams and ointments, on the other hand, can actually make matters worse. Avoid hydrocortisone creams and consult your healthcare provider before using over-the-counter products.

• Take good care of yourself. You need rest, good nutrition, and relaxation to get well fast. Having herpes may raise some emotional issues that cause additional stress; try to put these worries on hold. The bottom line is that you're sick and you will get better soon. It may be easier to tackle some of the emotional issues a little later.

Both medically and psychologically, the first episode is in many ways the toughest challenge that HSV poses. Getting through it in the most positive way requires a variety of resources. These include competent and sensitive medical care and solid factual information.

Beyond everything else, it's crucial to remember that the first episode is most likely the worst that HSV can throw your way.

MANAGING HERPES

5

RECURRENT GENITAL HERPES: THE LONG RUN

"It was about two months after my first episode," says Leslie. "Things were pretty much back to normal in my life, and I was hoping that I wouldn't have any more trouble with this. One week I was working late a lot and having trouble sleeping. I ended up feeling kind of run-down. I don't know if this was related, but a couple of days later, the herpes came back.

"I remember being really upset about that second outbreak, and obsessing about it, checking myself all the time. That probably made matters worse, but even so, the sores lasted less than a week. And other than some itchiness, I felt fine.

"It turned out that I had about four or five outbreaks that first year, all pretty much the same. I didn't do anything special about them, because they weren't that much of a bother. Later the outbreaks got milder, but I still had about the same number each year."

If you're in the midst of a first episode, the very word recurrent may give you a feeling of dread. The prospect of going through this again is not a happy one. But don't think the worst: Recurrences of genital herpes are usually very different from first episodes and much less troublesome.

While Leslie's story is a familiar one, the specifics change for every individual. You may have only one or two herpes flare-ups in your whole life. You may have one or two each year. In some years, you may have a great many more. What happens in each case depends largely on a number of variables. Most, like the genetic make-up of your particular immune system or the strain of virus you were infected with, are completely beyond your control. But some you can influence by the way you manage your health.

LATENCY

To understand the mechanism of recurrent herpes, let's discuss further the ability of herpes simplex virus (HSV) and other herpesviruses to hide away and persist in the body. Immediately after infection with HSV, a person may experience signs of illness (first episode) or may have no symptoms at all. Either way, the immune system will attack HSV and eventually force the virus to retreat.

Specifically, after the initial episode of genital herpes, HSV will move away from the skin surface and travel along the nerve pathways to the sacral ganglia, the nerve roots that lie near the base of the spine. There, it goes into an inactive phase. As we explained in Chapter 2, the virus' ability to hide in this way and establish a permanent presence is called latency. During its inactive phase, HSV does not make more copies of itself (replicate) or move within the body. One analogy might be an army that retreats to a safe place and sets up a base camp. HSV's base camp in the ganglia is safe from the surveillance of the immune system.

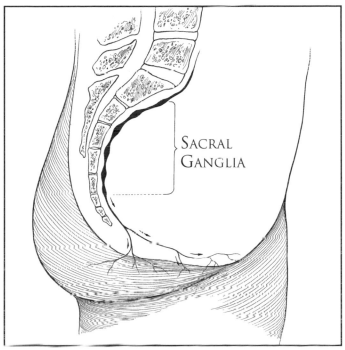

FIGURE 4. *When activated, HSV travels the nerve pathways back to the skin surface. Reactivation can cause the virus to reach the skin or mucosal membranes at many different sites in the genital area.*

REACTIVATION

When latent HSV does become active, it begins to replicate. To take our army metaphor further, we might think of active phases as times when the army will send out raiding parties to travel the nerve pathways towards the skin. Here the army becomes vulnerable to detection and counterattack, but it always has its base camp when it retreats.

Traveling the pathways of the nervous system in its active phase, HSV returns to the surface of the skin. There it can cause an outbreak—ulcers, sores, bumps, or other symptoms of genital herpes. This is often called *symptomatic* herpes, meaning that either the patient or the healthcare provider has some physical evidence that HSV is again stirring up trouble. The medical literature uses the term *viral shedding* to denote the presence of active virus on a skin or mucous membrane surface during these times.

Latent herpes simplex also can become active and travel the nerve pathways *without* causing signs and symptoms of illness. In the medical literature, this phenomenon has been called a number of things, including *asymptomatic viral shedding* and *subclinical shedding*. Here, when we use the term *asymptomatic shedding,* we mean the presence of virus on the skin or mucous membranes in the absence of symptoms. (In strict usage, *symptoms* refers to any marker of disease —including not only visible lesions but subjective feelings such as burning or itching. Therefore a person who experiences itching, for example, *would not* be asymptomatic.)

RECURRENCES WITH SYMPTOMS

Cases in which reactivation causes sores or other skin lesions are usually called *recurrences* or simply *outbreaks.* Here we will use the two terms interchangeably.

Most people who have a symptomatic first episode will have recurrences. With recurrences, people may experience a wide range of symptoms, some of them very subtle. As with first episodes, there are certain classic symptoms worth mentioning.

STAGES OF RECURRENT GENITAL HERPES AND
THREE POSSIBLE PRESENTATIONS

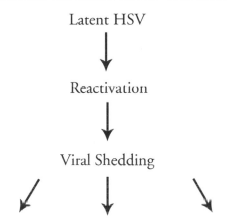

Latent HSV

Reactivation

Viral Shedding

1. No signs or symptoms   2. Prodrome; mild symptoms   3. Classic lesions

Prodrome

First, many people notice an itching, tingling, or burning sensation in the genital area before they see any visible signs of illness. These sensations are called the *prodrome*, and they can serve as a kind of early alarm system, warning that an outbreak may be on the way. Prodrome involves irritation along the nerves affected by HSV. Because nerve pathways connect in complicated patterns, this kind of irritation may lead to pain in the buttocks or the legs. The prodrome can last for several days but usually lasts less than 24 hours.

Other Signs and Symptoms

The prodrome is often followed by soreness or tenderness in a specific place, which in turn gives way to redness or skin irritation.

Next, in many cases, ulcers or small blisters form on the skin. These can follow the same stages of healing described in Chapter 4, but fortunately, the lesions seen in a recurrence are usually fewer in number and heal more quickly. Studies report an average healing time of 4 to 6 days for untreated recurrences. Women tend to have more painful symptoms than men in recurrent herpes, but people of either sex very seldom have generalized symptoms such as fever, malaise, or fatigue.

Recurrent herpes usually affects the external genitals, less commonly reaching internal surfaces such as the cervix or the urethra. For example, recurrences produce evidence of virus on the cervix in only 12% of women, not the rate of up to 80% found in first-episode genital herpes.

We've already stressed that symptoms can vary a great deal from person to person. They can also change within an individual from one outbreak to the next, and certainly can change greatly over long periods of time.

Genital herpes can cause very minor signs and symptoms that are easy to overlook or, as we mentioned in Chapter 4, may be confused with other ailments. Herpes lesions may be as subtle as a pimple, a small break in the skin, or a tiny area of redness. Sometimes herpes sores look like small linear fissures and are mistaken for a yeast infection. Sometimes they may fall at the site of a hair follicle and be mistaken for an ingrown hair. Another example is minor lesions around the rectum, which are hard to see and are commonly mistaken for hemorrhoids. Not only are many of the signs and symptoms of herpes subtle, but they frequently clear up quickly as well, perhaps taking only a day or two to disappear. Not infrequently, people experience prodrome and then have no lesions at all.

The wide variety of symptoms is the major reason that a visual diagnosis isn't always reliable. Illustrating the diverse symptoms and potential confusion associated with genital herpes, the table below was compiled by researchers at the Virology Research Clinic of the University of Washington. Patients presenting to the clinic with the initial complaints listed below were in fact diagnosed with genital herpes.

It's also worth noting that genital herpes symptoms don't always show up in the same place. A man might experience lesions on the penis the first several times he has an outbreak, for example, and then discover herpes lesions on his buttock or upper thigh the next time. Overall, about 20% of people will have a non-genital herpes recurrence, and the buttocks and legs are the most likely sites for such recurrences.

People sometimes find that the site of their outbreaks changes over time, and they worry that the virus might show up anywhere.

GENITAL HERPES SYMPTOMS MAY BE CONFUSED WITH...

IN WOMEN		IN MEN	
Yeast infection	Allergy to...	Folliculitis	Irritation from...
Vaginitis	• condoms	Jock itch	• tight jeans
	• spermicide		• sexual
Urinary tract infection	• spermicide	"Normal" itching	intercourse
		Zipper burn	• bicycle seat
Menstruation	Irritation from...		
	• bicycle seat	Hemorrhoids	
Hemorrhoids	• shaving		
	• douching	Allergy to condoms	
Heat rash		Insect or spider bite	
Urethral syndrome			

It won't. A genital herpes infection is limited by the nerve pathways connected to the sacral ganglion. With genital HSV, signs and symptoms may migrate a few inches here or there, but they will remain in the same general area, below the waist. As noted earlier, there are instances in which herpes sores develop on the face, for example, during or after a troublesome first episode. These sores may result from

The skin lesions of genital herpes vary in appearance as well as in location. The following illustrations offer just a few examples of common sites for herpes recurrences. Lesions often are more subtle than those shown here. Because lesions may be located in the perineal or perianal area, or on the inner thigh, they may be difficult to see.

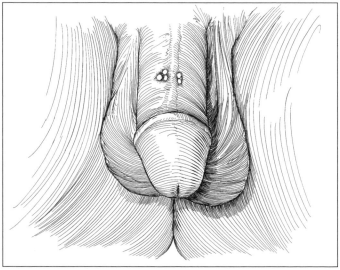

FIGURE 5. *Fluid filled blisters on the shaft of the penis, consistent with recurrent genital herpes.*

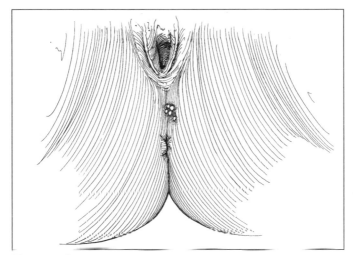

FIGURE 6. *Herpes lesions in the perineal area.*

FIGURE 7. *Herpes lesions on the buttocks near the anus.*

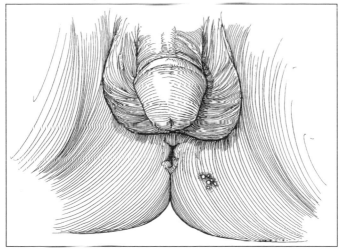

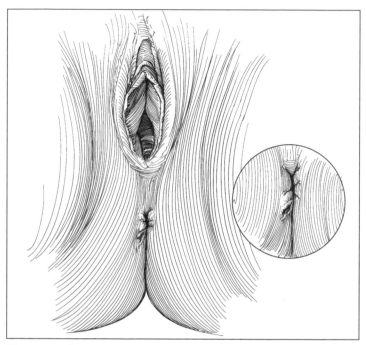

FIGURE 8. *A slight fissure (slit) near the anus. This is a common site for herpes lesions, which are sometimes mistaken for hemorrhoids.*

autoinoculation; more commonly, though, they occur because a person has had a prior oral herpes infection. Don't jump to the conclusion that genital herpes has packed up and moved to the face on its own.

Post-Herpetic Neuralgia

One further note on symptoms: A small number of people with genital herpes report pain or discomfort in the general area of

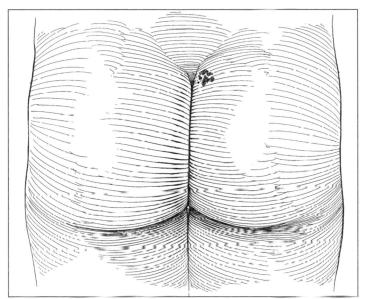

FIGURE 9. *Lesions of genital herpes on the buttocks. These are often thought to be "spider bites." They are sometimes misdiagnosed by healthcare providers as herpes zoster (shingles).*

the healed lesions after the normal symptoms of a recurrence have ended. The term sometimes applied to this condition is *post-herpetic neuralgia,* meaning pain that extends along the course of one or more nerves. Post-herpetic neuralgia is frequently experienced by people with shingles (caused by the varicella zoster virus), and has been studied best in that population. Unfortunately, however, there is very little research on HSV-related neuralgia. The frequency of this complication remains unknown, and there are no widely accepted guidelines on treatment.

43

Based on what's known about shingles, people experiencing pain or discomfort following a herpes outbreak should regard HSV as being in its active phase during this time. Analgesics such as aspirin or ibuprofen are probably the most basic remedies available for the pain, but the antiviral medications discussed in Chapter 9 may help to reduce the duration of post-herpetic neuralgia. Antivirals have been shown to reduce the duration of post-lesion pain in shingles patients by 50% or more. For people in whom post-herpetic neuralgia is linked with frequent recurrences of genital herpes, there may be value in using a daily antiviral medication to suppress the outbreaks and thereby lessen the problem of repeated irritation to the nerves.

How Likely Are Recurrences?

It's difficult to predict the pattern of recurrences in any individual case. There are, in fact, some people who never have anything resembling a classic herpes outbreak. The latest research suggests that as few as 15% of those with antibodies to HSV-2 recognize the infection—that is, when asked if they have ever had genital herpes, they say no. One would be tempted to assume, then, these persons do not have noticeable, recurrent symptoms. As we explained in Chapter 4, however, recent studies have shown that many of them do. In one such study, among a group of individuals who tested positive for HSV-2 but were unaware of their infection, roughly 70% learned to recognize recurrent symptoms after being educated about herpes by the research team. The bottom line: Most people with HSV-2 antibodies do have symptoms they can learn to recognize as herpes. In some cases, these might be marked outbreaks; in others, they might be minor irritations that could easily be overlooked.

These are large generalizations, taking into account all the millions of people for whom herpes symptoms will never be bothersome enough to spur a trip to the healthcare provider. But the experts have more specific information when it comes to people whose first episode brought noticeable symptoms. Because these people often seek medical care, researchers have been able to run studies in which the patients are monitored for many years, leading to several important observations.

Viral Type Matters: Understanding Sites of Preference

Whether and how often you have recurrences depends to a great extent on which type of HSV you have. If your primary episode is caused by HSV-1, for example, there is a 50% to 60% chance you will have a recurrence in the first year. By contrast, if the primary episode is caused by HSV-2, the chance of a symptomatic recurrence in the first year is 90%. And perhaps more important, people with genital HSV-2 are likely to have not just one but several recurrences in this and following years.

Why is this? Researchers don't fully understand it, but they know that type 1 and type 2 have definite *sites of preference*. Scientists suppose that each viral type is triggered by certain events or chain reactions that may be specific to the body site where they're found.

In any case, HSV-1 causes the overwhelming majority of oral-facial herpes, and a person with HSV-1 latent in the facial area is much more likely to have recurrent outbreaks on the face than a person with HSV-2 in the same place. Today, HSV-1 accounts for an increasing percentage of genital herpes infections—up to 50% depending upon the population studied. In addition, a first episode caused by HSV-1 is just as severe as that caused by HSV-2. However, people with HSV-1 genital herpes are likely to have only a few outbreaks or none at all after the first episode is healed. The bottom line is that genital HSV-1 is likely to be largely quiescent after year 1.

The site of preference for HSV-2 is the genital area. Genital HSV-2 is very likely to cause multiple outbreaks, not only in year 1 but in later years as well. By contrast, it seldom causes symptoms above the waist (as an oral infection, for example).

Long-Term Patterns

As with predicting the likelihood of recurrences, predicting their number and long-term pattern is very hard. Do outbreaks become less frequent after five years? Ten years? Do they become less severe? While medical science doesn't have a way to predict the course of herpes for any particular individual, researchers have been studying genital herpes long enough to make some useful observations about long-term patterns of recurrence.

A study published in 1999, for example, analyzed the medical histories of 664 people with recurrent genital herpes over a period of 1 to 18 years. Consistent with earlier studies, this analysis showed that patients with HSV-1 had the lowest recurrence rates—a single recurrence on average in year one and a fraction of that in subsequent years. Patients with HSV-2, by contrast, had an average of five recurrences per year in the first year.

Of equal importance, the number of recurrences per year appears to decrease over time in the majority of patients. Overall, those who were enrolled in the study based on a first episode of HSV-2 and who were followed for more than 4 years had a median decrease of 2 recurrences per year between years 1 and 5. Thus, a person with 6 recurrences in year 1 would be having 4 recurrences after year 5, and a person with 4 recurrences in year 1 would be down to 2 outbreaks after year 5. Some 25% of the study subjects, however, actually experienced an *increase* of at least one recurrence per year, illustrating that herpes is highly variable from one person to the next.

Earlier studies reflected some of this variability as well, and it's impossible to predict where any given individual will fit into this game of averages. Among other observations made in long-term studies: Patients with longer lasting first episodes tend to have more frequent recurrences than those with milder first episodes.

REACTIVATION WITHOUT SYMPTOMS

For many years, scientists thought that HSV had basically two modes. One was the active phase, in which an infected person clearly had lesions or marked symptoms of some kind. The second was the inactive phase, in which HSV was out of the picture and of no consequence.

As they learned more about the virus, however, researchers discovered that HSV could become active and yet *cause no symptoms*—at least none the patient would be aware of. This phenomenon is the *asymptomatic* form of herpes described earlier in this chapter.

With truly asymptomatic herpes, there is neither discomfort nor a lesion that the patient can see, so we might be tempted to write it off as irrelevant. But when virus travels to skin sites or to mucous membranes, there is the possibility of *viral shedding*, which creates a risk of spreading herpes to others during sexual contact.

There are still unanswered questions about asymptomatic viral shedding, but much has been learned in the last few years. Researchers have studied people who have visible symptoms from time to time, asking them to test themselves daily between outbreaks. In these studies, several observations seem fairly consistent:

• Asymptomatic shedding occurs in the vast majority of people who have and recognize recurrent genital herpes and in people who are HSV-2 seropositive but may not have recognized genital symptoms. There is variability in shedding rates. For some people it happens on a small percentage of days—perhaps less than 20 days over the course of a year. For others it may occur much more often. The average is about 13% of days per year.

• The amount of virus present is similar to what is found during symptomatic outbreaks, and it's often sufficient to spread the infection to a partner.

• The amount of asymptomatic shedding is greatest in the first year after one acquires genital HSV-2—roughly twice as high as in year two.

• As with symptomatic recurrences, asymptomatic shedding is more than three times as frequent in those with genital HSV-2 as in those with genital HSV-1.

• The risk of asymptomatic shedding exists in everyone with genital herpes. While the frequency varies from person to person, someone with mild disease may shed as much virus as a person with severe infection.

• Asymptomatic shedding can occur almost anywhere in the genital region. As with all HSV reactivation, the virus follows the nerve pathways connected to the ganglion at the base of the spine. Especially likely sites of shedding, however, are the vulva and perianal area in women or the shaft of the penis and perianal area in men.

In summary, what's most remarkable about asymptomatic shedding is that it appears to follow the major patterns associated with recognized outbreaks: It occurs in almost everyone with genital HSV-2; it's more likely with HSV-2 than HSV-1; and it produces quantities of virus sufficient to cause transmission.

What about those who are diagnosed on the basis of a blood test but have no history of symptoms—how often do they shed virus? Research on viral shedding in those with no history of symptoms is a relatively new undertaking, but some observations can be made based on a study published in 2000. In this study, 53 persons with no history of recurrences were educated about herpes, asked to perform daily swabs of the genital area for laboratory testing, and followed closely by clinic staff for just over three months. Results from this group were then compared with 90 subjects who had a history of genital herpes recurrences. Analysis showed the following:

• Eighty-three percent of those who gave no history were found to have viral shedding during the study.

• After education and counseling, 80% had and were able to recognize a symptomatic recurrence during follow-up.

• Those with no history of symptoms had 60% fewer symptomatic recurrences, and their recurrences were 40% shorter on average than those experienced by subjects in the other group.

• Overall rates of viral shedding (including both outbreaks and days with asymptomatic shedding) were lower in the group with no history, with virus present according to a viral culture test on 3.8% of days, versus 6.4% in the symptomatic group.

• Rates of asymptomatic shedding were similar in both groups.

All in all, only one person in this group of 58 had neither a recognized outbreak nor a documented episode of viral shedding. What these findings suggest is that those who have HSV-2 as measured by a blood test but never recognize any symptoms do, in fact, have phases in which HSV becomes active and causes viral shedding. In this group, however, most of these active phases take the form of asymptomatic shedding rather than outbreaks. Asymptomatic shedding accounts for about one-third of all reactivation in those with recognized outbreaks and roughly 80% of shedding in those with more subtle infections, so it's important to understand it. Researchers already have established that asymptomatic shedding, as well as shedding during recurrences, can be suppressed in part with medication. This is covered in Chapter 9.

WHAT TRIGGERS RECURRENCES?

Long-term patterns in the cycle of active and inactive phases also raise the question: What triggers HSV to break out of its dormant phase and become active again? Can outbreaks be avoided simply by avoiding these triggers?

Over the years, people with herpes have put forth many candidates as the trigger for recurrences. These include sickness, psychological stress, fatigue, menstruation, and poor nutrition. Sun exposure—even the mildest sunburn—can be a trigger for HSV, as can irritation or friction at the site of infection. And some say that vigorous sex can cause this kind of irritation.

Few of these possible triggers have been closely studied by researchers, but some work has been done. Scientists have noted several types of outbreak stimulants in lab animals, among them: Radiation, skin irritation at the site of infection, and surgical trauma to the nerve or ganglion where the latent virus resides.

Recently, very detailed studies have looked at the role of intense ultraviolet light on facial cold sores caused by HSV-1. In these studies, 70% of the subjects exposed to about two hours of midday sun developed herpes symptoms within a week. Subjects who used sunscreen were protected. The message for people who get cold sores is clear, particularly if they're sensitive to the sun. On the basis of a few small research studies, it seems that ultraviolet light may have a similar effect in triggering genital herpes.

Menstruation remains prominent as a trigger factor in anecdotal accounts, but researchers have found no evidence of this in research studies.

Psychological stress has received a great deal of attention as a possible trigger factor. Over two-thirds of the respondents in ASHA's 1991 survey, for example, indicated that "stressful events contribute to herpes symptoms." This issue also has been examined by a variety of researchers, with somewhat contradictory results. The latest study on stress, published in 1999, suggests that there is not a relationship between short-term stress—say, a deadline at the office—and genital herpes recurrences. There was, however, a slight increase in risk of a recurrence associated with stressors lasting more than 7 days—for example, a period of anxiety about prolonged unemployment.

In any case, can you avoid triggers? From a strictly scientific point of view, outbreaks cannot be predicted with accuracy. No one will be able to identify the certain cause of every flare-up, and some people won't have a clue about any of them. At the same time, however, it appears that many people with herpes do begin to associate certain events or behaviors with reactivation.

Once identified, triggers can *sometimes* be avoided. If sunburn gives you a bad case of cold sores, there is always sunscreen, lip balm, and a hat. If outbreaks seem to be brought on by fatigue, maybe it's time to get serious about a quality eight hours of sleep every night.

Stress is perhaps a more troublesome category. There is little point for most of us in trying to create "stress-free" lives. In fact, even if we did, there is no proof that we'd be free from HSV reactivations. Nonetheless, it's widely accepted that managing stress through exercise or other activities can be beneficial to one's overall physical and mental health. It's possible, though not proven, that this may have some benefit in managing herpes as well.

Many triggers are not known or can't be foreseen. Others you may have good reason to suspect but can't do much about. The last thing you want to do is blame yourself for recurrences or try endless experimental strategies to avoid them. For some, this becomes another form of obsession.

If, on the other hand, you gain clear insight into your pattern of outbreaks, you may find practical ways of sometimes averting them. Over time your knowledge of your own triggers and your sensitivity to prodromal symptoms will likely increase. This information, in turn, is something you can use in a variety of ways, including taking preventive medications or taking precautions to lower the risk of transmitting herpes to a sexual partner.

THE BOTTOM LINE

The next few chapters of this book offer many ideas on how to manage recurrent genital herpes. But there are a number of points we've already covered that are worth emphasizing:

• Viral type is the most important factor influencing the course of recurrent genital herpes. Therefore, it's important to know which type you have. Chapter 16 explains which diagnostic tests provide this information.

• Statistical data show that those with HSV-2 typically have several recurrences per year while those with HSV-1 have few or none. However, there is great variability between individuals. Some people have only a few outbreaks each year, while others have many. The pattern is different for everyone.

• The symptoms caused by herpes outbreaks may change over time. Sores might appear in one spot this month and several inches away three months from now. Some outbreaks may simply result in irritation or redness.

• Outbreaks are not the only concern with genital herpes. There are times when HSV reactivates in the form of asymptomatic viral shedding, and one can be contagious at these times. Like recurrences, asymptomatic shedding tends to be more frequent in the first year and more frequent in those with HSV-2.

• There is little hard evidence about what triggers out

breaks, but a great many people report that they associate certain stresses or behaviors with outbreaks.

6

HOW IS HERPES SPREAD?

"I was just diagnosed with herpes," says a caller to the National Herpes Hotline. "And I'm worried about giving this thing to someone else. I'm confused about how I got it, and I don't really know when I'm contagious."

Understanding how the herpes simplex virus (HSV) operates and what you can expect it to do inside your body are crucial pieces of information. But equally pressing is the issue of *transmission.* People want to know how they got infected with herpes—when, and by whom, and in what precise way. They also wonder when they're contagious.

This is one of the most complex aspects of herpes and one that usually takes a bit of study to grasp fully. It may be necessary to read this chapter and the next a few times before the information makes complete sense or before you can remember it all.

The first basic rule is that genital herpes spreads from one person to another through various forms of sexual intimacy, all of them involving direct body-to-body contact. We'll talk about these in more detail on the following pages.

Second, the possibility that herpes will be spread from one person to another exists only at times when there is viral shedding—

times when HSV is present on a skin surface or mucous membrane.

As we discussed in Chapters 4 and 5, active periods of viral shedding are often marked by signs or symptoms—either classic herpes lesions or the more subtle presentations that are easily confused with other ailments. It's also possible that the viral shedding caused by an active phase will be entirely *asymptomatic* and that you will be totally unaware of it. This scenario will be covered more fully later in this chapter (see the section titled, "When No Symptoms Are Present").

The most flagrant sign that herpes has become active is the presence of sores or some kind of lesion on the surface of the skin. We'll address this issue first.

WHEN SYMPTOMS ARE PRESENT

As an example, let's say you have two or three herpes sores on your genitals during your first recurrence. The sores are, in effect, little colonies of virus, and as long as you can see them, you should assume you have significant amounts of HSV present on the surface of the skin. If you have sexual intercourse while the sores are present, it's likely that your partner's genitals will come in direct contact with these sores. That would give the virus a chance to spread to your partner's skin and take up residence there.

The risk of infecting another person begins with the itching or tingling feeling that you get right before an outbreak. If you notice any symptoms of recurrent genital herpes—even the prodrome— take it as a sign that the virus has found its way to the skin or to the mucous membranes usually affected. The risk continues as long as you notice *any* kind of symptom. If sores or other skin lesions are present, it's best to consider these contagious until they have completely healed. The tender new skin you see after a scab falls off might not be contagious, but caution is advisable: Asymptomatic shedding is more likely to occur within the first few days before and after an outbreak than at other times. Herpes can be spread through other forms of direct skin-to-skin contact as well. Consider what can happen during oral sex. When a person with a cold sore on the lips has oral contact with a partner's genitals, the virus has an opportunity. Herpes can spread from the lips to the partner's genitals, causing genital herpes.

The direct contact that occurs during oral sex also can cause an infection in the facial area. Let's say a person engages in oral sex with a partner who has herpes sores on the genitals. Contact with those genital sores can give the virus a chance to spread to the person's lips or mouth, resulting in herpes infection in the facial area.

Sexual intimacy provides several possible ways in which active virus may have a chance to spread from a site of viral shedding to susceptible genital tissue or mucous membrane in a partner. We've specifically mentioned oral-genital sex. Other routes of transmission include penile-vaginal intercourse, penetration of the anus, and oral-anal contact. Even the rubbing of one body against another without penetration might give active virus a chance to spread, assuming the uninfected person is exposing susceptible skin in the genital area.

All of this can be a little confusing. People sometimes ask, for instance, "Now that I've got genital herpes, does it mean the virus is going to migrate all over my body and trigger cold sores on the lips?" They wonder if they're going to be spreading herpes when they touch someone or kiss someone. The answer to all of these questions is no. Herpes simplex will not relocate from your genital area to your facial area or any other part of your body unless you give it a lot of help. It can be spread from the genitals to a sexual partner's face in the way we have described, but it doesn't get up and move all by itself.

Remember the rule of thumb: Herpes is spread through direct skin-to-skin contact with an area where virus is active on the skin.

Non-Genital and Non-Mucosal Sites

You may be wondering why herpes seems to take hold only in the genital region or around the mouth. HSV has evolved to thrive in warm and moist environments, and genital skin like that of the vulva or penis offers the virus a suitable entryway. So do soft, moist mucosal surfaces such as the vagina, cervix, anus, and mouth. The thicker, tougher skin on the arms and legs, by contrast, is generally not hospitable to HSV. If by chance HSV is deposited on these parts of the body, it usually withers before it has a chance to find the nerve pathways and go about the complex business of making its permanent home.

Notice the word 'usually' in the last sentence. There are some cases where herpes does penetrate the tough skin of the hands or the chest, for example. But in these instances the process of transmission is helped along by some damage to the skin in question.

A good illustration of this principle is an HSV infection called *herpes gladiatorum*—what some call *wrestler's herpes*. In a number of cases, high school or college wrestlers have developed herpes sores on the chest or arms in the aftermath of a wrestling tournament. Why? Wrestling involves rolling around on the mat and grabbing the arms and torso of the opponent, all of which can be abrasive to the skin—even thick skin. Add to this the fact that wrestlers spend a good deal of time in tight embraces, and you can see that direct contact with a cold sore (or with saliva that contains HSV from oral herpes) might give HSV a chance to spread from one wrestler to another.

This happens only rarely, and the circumstances under which it

has occurred sometimes involve a wrestler who is particularly contagious because he is having a first episode of type 1 herpes on the face.
During this kind of outbreak, large amounts of virus might be present on the surface of the skin or in saliva, and lesions on the face are
not uncommon.

Another scenario in which herpes can spread to thicker skin is
autoinoculation. As described in Chapter 2, this occurs when someone touches a herpes sore—on the genitals, let's say—and then ends
up sometime later with a herpes outbreak on the finger, usually
around the nail bed, as the virus is most likely to enter the damaged skin in that area. The route of transmission is clear. Active virus
from a sore found its way to the finger when the person touched or
scratched the sore. The virus then managed to find some portal of
entry—a cut or scrape, for example—so that it could travel the nerve
pathways and set up shop in a different location, such as moving
from the genitals to a finger. Autoinoculation seems to be most common when the site of new infection is another mucous membrane.
(Sometimes people get herpes sores in or around the eyes, a subject
discussed in Chapter 16.)

To keep this in proper perspective, don't forget that autoinoculation is relatively infrequent. It occurs almost exclusively during first
episodes, when there are lots of sores and an unusually high dose of
virus on the skin. It's estimated that autoinoculation occurs in about
10% of first episodes, but it's rare with recurrent genital herpes.
The reason is that within a few months the body develops a strong
immune response to the virus.

To sum up, the best advice is to regard the presence of prodrome,
sores, or any potentially herpes-related lesion as a sign that the virus
is active and could be spread. Any kind of direct skin-to-skin contact
with the sores or lesions creates a risk for the spread of the virus, but

it's almost always *sexual* contact—genital-to-genital, oral-to-genital, or oral-to-oral contact—that causes new infections.

WHEN NO SYMPTOMS ARE PRESENT

Unfortunately, the HSV's active phase is not always marked by the presence of signs and symptoms. Chapter 5 describes the phenomenon of asymptomatic shedding, in which herpes reactivates and travels to the skin without setting off the usual alarm system. It's now clear from a number of studies that herpes can be spread at these times, in a process called *asymptomatic transmission.*

These are troublesome facts of life for people with herpes, because they complicate the issue of protecting a sexual partner from infection. Even those who don't recall ever having had symptoms face this risk of giving the infection to a partner. Nevertheless, there are a number of ways to approach this problem of asymptomatic herpes, and the best way to begin is by understanding more about how it works.

In a general sense, asymptomatic shedding is somewhat similar to regular outbreaks: While herpes is in its latent phase, some event triggers a recurrence. HSV travels through the nerve pathways to the area where it usually causes symptoms, and finds its way to the surface of the skin or to a mucous membrane such as the cervix. Meanwhile, the immune system comes into play and thwarts the virus, stopping HSV's spread before any major lesions appear—but unfortunately *not* before there is risk of transmission.

Where is asymptomatic shedding likely to occur? In most cases, HSV can be expected to travel the same routes it does during a symptomatic flare-up, and virus might reach the skin anywhere in the genital area, including the sites where you normally have signs and symptoms during a noticeable outbreak. In particular, asymptomatic shedding is likely on the vulva and perianal area in women, and the shaft of the penis and the perianal area in men.

Answering *when* shedding will occur is much more difficult. Just as with the question of what triggers outbreaks, the causes of asymptomatic shedding remain a bit of a riddle for scientists. Presumably the same mechanism is responsible for both types of reactivation.

Frequency of shedding, however, is somewhat better understood. As discussed in the previous chapter, patterns of asymptomatic shedding mimic recurrences in a number of ways. Asymptomatic shedding is highest in the first year after acquiring herpes, and in general, rates decline slightly over time. Just as recurrence rates vary greatly between individuals, so does asymptomatic shedding. This has been measured over the years in a long list of studies, many of which require patients to swab themselves daily in order to detect the presence of HSV. In the early years of these studies, the standard test was viral culture; in more recent years, the test of choice has been the much more sensitive PCR (polymerase chain reaction) assay, which can detect a minute number of virus particles. Shedding rates vary widely with each method used. By culture, for example, representative rates of shedding range from only 1% of days (3.6 days per year) to 15% of days. The average is approximately 4%. By PCR, the numbers run from 1% up to about 60%, with an average in the range of 13%.

These numerical values for viral shedding may be a useful guidepost, but the more compelling issue is transmission. It's clear that there is no risk of transmission without viral shedding, but researchers do not really know precisely how much shedding is required for transmission, nor do they understand all of the various factors that contribute to the spread of herpes.

Researchers have found antiviral therapy has basically the same effect on asymptomatic shedding that it does on outbreaks. In particular, a daily dose of suppressive therapy with acyclovir or valacyclovir reduces viral shedding by 90% when measured by culture and 70% when measured by PCR. A clinical study has shown that valacyclovir can lower the actual risk of transmission to partners, with a reduction in transmission risk of 48%. The role of medication will be discussed in depth in Chapter 9.

Whatever the actual rate in your case, the hard part is that you won't know which days these will be. So when it comes to protecting a sexual partner, this is an issue that requires you to talk things through and make certain decisions as a couple.

OTHER ISSUES FOR TRANSMISSION OF HSV

An important concern for couples who would like to have a child is the issue of managing herpes during pregnancy and birth. In some cases, HSV is transmitted to a baby at the time of delivery if the mother has active herpes in the birth canal at delivery. This is a very rare event among the tens of millions of women who have genital herpes, and there are well-known precautions that can prevent it in most cases. All the same, herpes infections in a newborn can be life-threatening, and expectant parents often have very specific questions about what they need to do to ensure a healthy birth. They also wonder about the risk to an infant in the home if one or both parents have recurrent oral or genital herpes. We've attempted to answer these questions in detail in Chapter 14.

Another frequent question centers on the spread of herpes from *things* rather than from people. Can you get herpes from a toilet seat, for example, or a dirty towel? The basic answer on the risk of getting herpes from inanimate objects like these is something along the lines of "generally impossible." The main reason for this goes back to our earlier discussion about transmission, about skin-to-skin contact, and about the likely places where herpes can take hold. If you rubbed a herpes sore against a towel, for instance, some of the herpes simplex virus could be deposited onto the towel. The virus may persist outside the body for several hours, but soon it begins to lose its ability to invade and colonize new cells.

Now take the example of the toilet seat and follow the rules of transmission. In order to spread herpes, a person has to be infected, to have active herpes, and to have virus present on the skin. Furthermore, the skin in question would have to come into contact with the surface of the toilet seat. Since people generally do not rub their genitals against toilet seats, a person would have to have active herpes on the back of the thigh or lower buttock in order to place virus on the seat. This is not the most likely place to have an outbreak.

Next, within a short time, a second person would have to sit on the same seat, making contact with the seat in exactly the same spot, thereby coming into contact with HSV. And would the virus find a hospitable environment there on the back of the thigh? Probably not. The skin there is thick, making it an unlikely target.

Often, the context for questions about non-sexual transmission of herpes is the concern about parent-child transmission in the household. For example, a mother has a history of herpes and worries about diapering her three-month-old baby or getting in the tub with a one-year-old. What is the chance that herpes will be spread from parent to child over the course of many years of casual household contact—from diapering to sharing towels? Frankly, these questions do not have clear-cut answers based on scientific data. However, there is not a single published case of HSV transmission via an inanimate object, and the most logical conclusions to draw from this fact is that casual household transmission is extremely rare or nonexistent.

Researchers, however, do acknowledge a *theoretical* risk of non-sexual transmission. A damp towel shared by two people showering together, for example, could hypothetically provide a means for the spread of herpes to the genitals if one person were having an outbreak and rubbed the towel on the site of infection before passing it to the partner.

Experts disagree about whether herpes is ever *really* spread in this way, but because it's theoretically possible, common sense dictates precautions. During active phases, don't share towels, underwear, or other objects that come into contact with herpes sores. In cases of facial herpes, the items to avoid sharing during active phases would be cups, toothbrushes, and razors. And if you touch a herpes lesion with your finger, take the precaution of washing your hands right away. Soapy water kills the virus.

PEOPLE WITH HERPES are likely to have a number of worries about spreading the infection to other people. It's natural to have these concerns. But sometimes people will become obsessed with risks that are either very remote or completely nonexistent. So, to put things in perspective, here are some overall guidelines.

• The greatest risk for spreading herpes comes when you have a herpes symptom—no matter how slight—and your partner's skin comes into direct contact with that area during sex. Avoiding this kind of contact is the first concern.

• If you have recurrent genital herpes, you will want to talk with your partner about the risk of asymptomatic transmission when you have sex during the times between outbreaks. See Chapter 13 for a full discussion of the different approaches that people take to prevent the spread of herpes in sexual relationships.

• If you're having your first-ever outbreak of genital herpes (or facial herpes), it's wise to be extra-cautious about hygiene. Avoid touching herpes sores, and if you do touch them, wash your hands right away with soap and water. Soap will kill the virus.

• If you are pregnant and you or your partner has a history of genital herpes, it's very important to inform your physician or midwife about this part of your medical history. If genital herpes becomes active at the time of delivery, your provider may need to take special precautions to protect your baby. This is discussed at length in Chapter 14.

• If you have a newborn in the household, take care to see that the child does not come in direct contact with herpes lesions. It isn't wise, for example, to kiss *anyone* if you have a cold sore on the mouth, but this is an especially important rule with infants.

The most critical issues for preventing transmission of HSV center on your sexual relationships. These will likely be among your leading concerns as you adjust to life with the herpes simplex virus.

7

WHO'S TO BLAME?

"It was a mystery," says Julia. "I remember being diagnosed with herpes and wondering where I got it. I didn't have a clue. I hadn't slept with anyone in months. So I called the two people I'd been with, and both said they'd never had herpes. They thanked me for telling them about it. That was it. I never figured it out. And I never knew if I gave herpes to anyone else. I still wonder."

If you've just experienced your first outbreak of genital herpes— or if you were diagnosed on the basis of a blood test—you, too, may be asking the question: Where did I get this?

Given that genital herpes is a sexually transmitted infection, it's natural for people to scrutinize their current sexual relationships in search of an answer. Often they seek to blame a current partner for infecting them, especially if it's someone they've known only briefly. If they have been intimate with one person for a long time, they sometimes come to believe that this partner has recently had an affair, developed herpes as a result, and kept it a secret. Whatever the scenario, suspicion and anger are common elements, and they're often directed at a person's current lover.

Are these suspicions likely to be well-founded? It is possible to get a genital herpes infection from one's current sexual partner, but this is not always the correct explanation. Julia's story doesn't offer enough detail for even an educated guess, but with a little room for embellishment we can suggest at least three possible scenarios:

'It Had To Be You'

Julia is single and dating, having recently broken off a relationship of two years with Jim. She's currently seeing Mark off and on, and two months ago she slept with him a few times. Later she developed a genital rash and went to the healthcare provider who now has diagnosed her with genital herpes.

Can Julia legitimately blame Mark? The circumstantial evidence is fairly compelling, but in this example Julia actually had acquired herpes from her earlier boyfriend, Jim. Neither of them knew he had it, because he was one of those many millions who carry HSV-2 and never realize it. She never knew she had gotten it, because she had no obvious symptoms when she was first infected.

Now, over a year later, something has triggered a reactivation of the latent HSV. Julia has symptoms, and she's blaming Mark.

'It Had To Be Infidelity'

Let's keep two of the players, but change the details of the story:

Julia has been living with Mark for almost a year. She gets genital herpes symptoms and is diagnosed with it. She wants to blame Mark and so confronts him.

Mark says he doesn't have herpes—never had any STI or anything vaguely resembling herpes. Just as Julia suspects him, Mark now begins to suspect her. He knows that he hasn't been intimate with anyone else for more than a year. Now suddenly he is accused of having herpes. So he wonders if Julia has recently had an affair, has picked up this infection, and is simply afraid to admit it.

Well, Mark is wrong. It turns out that Mark does have herpes and did infect Julia. It's just that he didn't know he had it. He's one of those people who has very mild and infrequent symptoms, and he has never considered that they were related to an STI. For all practical purposes, he's being completely honest and above-board. But he does have genital herpes. And now Julia does, too.

'A LONG STORY'

Let's try one more variation:

Having broken off a relationship with Jim a year ago, Julia moves in with Mark. Two months later Julia comes back from the doctor with a diagnosis of genital herpes. She blames Mark; Mark blames her. Accusations of infidelity fly. Mark denies any history of herpes.

Then suddenly Mark, too, gets herpes. Julia is now fully convinced that she was right to blame him all along. Mark is equally convinced that Julia is at fault.

As in the first scenario, Julia actually had picked up herpes from her earlier relationship with Jim. But things have gotten really complicated now. Julia never knew she was infected until she just recently had her first outbreak. Meanwhile, she had infected Mark.

Everybody has herpes, and it all started with Jim.

IS REAL LIFE LIKE THIS? It isn't always, but it can be. These are actually fairly common scenarios.

If there is appeal in a guessing game, tracing genital herpes infection can be among the most challenging of mysteries. Countless people with herpes have puzzled over the spread of HSV and posed hard questions: How could this have happened to me? Are you sure it wasn't a toilet seat? Who was the culprit? Was my spouse unfaithful? Did my lover know he had herpes and keep it a secret from me?

For the most part, the questions cannot be answered. HSV, it turns out, is a very crafty virus. Trying to figure out how it spreads raises a host of complicated issues: Signs and symptoms, viral type, previous sexual history, prior infection with HSV, and so on.

The fictional scenarios presented here offer a glimpse at three critical reasons why it's hard to know who is to blame.

The first reason is that *you can have herpes and never know it.* Earlier chapters have gone into some detail about the evidence that up to 85% of all people diagnosed with HSV-2 infection based on screening tests say they have never had herpes symptoms. A small proportion of this group, as we've explained, probably are truly asymptomatic. Most, however, have mild symptoms they did not recognize as herpes. Either way, a large number of people get herpes and never know it, never think about it—never have any reason to talk about it or take precautions.

The second reason is that *you can get herpes and carry it around for months or years before you finally have a recognized outbreak.* Researchers believe that about one in four people seeking care for their first outbreak have actually had herpes for some time. It's possible to have a very mild first episode and to assume that it's something else—a yeast infection or an allergic rash, for example. Then, seemingly out of nowhere, the person with a mild or unrecognized infection can one day face a troublesome outbreak and wrongly assume that genital herpes is a new problem.

A third possible cause of confusion is that *you can spread herpes even when you don't have symptoms.* Studies have conclusively shown that persons infected with genital HSV have periodic episodes of asymptomatic viral shedding whether they have symptoms they recognize or not. So there are times when virus is present on the genital skin or mucous membranes. And that raises the possibility of spreading it to someone else during sexual contact. People who know they have genital herpes usually take some precautions to protect sexual partners, at least during known outbreaks. People who are unaware they have it, on the other hand, may see no reason to practice any form of risk reduction with their sexual partners.

Of course, asymptomatic transmission is a risk even for people with outbreaks that they do recognize as genital herpes. Sometimes a person might be careful to refrain from sex when symptoms are present and be unlucky enough to spread HSV to a partner during a period of viral shedding between outbreaks.

If all these hypotheticals seem a little overwhelming, be aware that this topic can be overwhelming for almost anyone—including skilled medical professionals. If you're trying to pinpoint the source of your herpes infection, you may well run into some dead ends. And it's likely that your healthcare provider won't be able to solve the mystery either.

Is there any way to know for sure? Can you get special tests that pinpoint the source? The path is not an easy one, but there are some facts you can probably establish with the help of a medical professional. With the right diagnostic test, for example, you may be able to determine whether or not you are having a first episode or a recurrence. The antibodies that a newly infected person produces to fight herpes usually will not be fully in evidence until some weeks after initial infection. Therefore, healthcare professionals can sometimes test for antibodies over a period of time to watch for a trend. A person newly infected with HSV-2 would have few or no antibodies to HSV-2 when blood was first drawn but would normally have a substantial level two to three months later.

Diagnosing a first episode versus a recurrence based on this evidence, however, is not as straightforward as it may seem here. Much depends on the specific signs and symptoms, the timing of the office visit, and the particular tests used to make the diagnosis. Some blood tests are useful for this type of detective work, and some are completely unreliable. It's possible that the test you want may not be available to you through your current healthcare provider or that the results will not be definitive. A detailed explanation of available tests will be coming in Chapter 16.

In any case, even if a blood test reveals that you are having a first episode, this evidence will not necessarily tell you *the source* of your herpes infection. As the fictional scenarios at the beginning of this chapter suggest, a lot depends on your own sexual history and a host of factors too complicated to explain in a book of this size. The moral is this: Don't be too quick to judge the situation. Figuring out the source of a herpes infection can stump even the best medical detective.

What's more, even if you are fairly sure about how you got herpes, it can be very wrong to assume that the partner in question was acting irresponsibly. There are indeed some people who know they have herpes and withhold this information from sexual partners. But there are many more who have no idea they themselves are infected, much less that they might be putting you at risk. In the end, understanding and forgiveness may give you more comfort than blame or vengefulness.

8

PATIENT AND PROVIDER

"The nurse practitioner who diagnosed me did a great job explaining all of this to me and helped to settle me down," says Barbara. "She seemed to know what the hot-button issues were and had lots of good information, including some excellent Web sites. I was presented with options for treatment right away and asked for my input. I could have used more time, but what I did get was quality."

For most people, the issue of getting the help they need begins with their healthcare provider. The provider is often the first person we ever talk to about genital herpes, and the tone and content of that conversation often shapes how we perceive herpes and how we manage it. Ideally, if you already have been diagnosed with genital herpes, your provider spent enough time with you to answer your questions about the herpes simplex virus, its likely pattern of recurrences, and the options available for treatment. If you had questions about how you got herpes, perhaps these were covered during the office visits, along with questions about your risk of spreading it to others. If so, you have an exceptional resource in your provider—a person you may be able to turn to as questions come up.

In many cases, however, people newly diagnosed with herpes report frustrations about their healthcare experiences. Even if you normally get along well with your healthcare provider, a diagnosis of genital herpes can complicate matters. It's important to be aware of some of the potentially tricky issues in order to continue a positive working relationship with your chosen medical professional.

If there are troubles, they often start with the visit in which herpes is diagnosed. The diagnosis itself is tough to hear and tough to deliver. And, depending on the individual, the diagnosis can raise several issues of importance to the patient. In all fairness, it's very difficult for healthcare providers to cover all of these issues in one visit. With a waiting room full of patients, there isn't time to say or do everything the provider would like to. Beyond this, providers may feel that they aren't prepared to discuss some of the emotional aspects of herpes.

From the patient's point of view, it's often devastating to learn that the illness at hand is caused by a sexually transmitted infection. Worse still, it's a viral infection and will stay with you for life. This news raises a great many questions about herpes itself and about its potential impact on important relationships.

The medical information alone is complex. The first several chapters of this book, for example, cover most of the basics. But how many healthcare professionals have the time to cover those topics on a first visit, especially if they haven't had the chance to schedule an extended session? Beyond this, patients can bring up emotional issues for which the healthcare professional may not have ready answers. "What will this mean for my sex life?" "How can I tell my lover?" Some of the questions cannot be answered in simple black and white.

From the provider's point of view, time and the patient's emotions are the most important constraints. Healthcare professionals often say they do their best to counsel patients on the key points but that patients' feelings of anger or disbelief sometimes stand in the way. A patient might be too upset to take in a lot of medical information—or might not remember many details later even if they were covered in a counseling session. Plus, with a waiting room full of patients, there isn't time to say or do everything the healthcare provider would like. Sometimes the best solution seems to be scheduling a follow-up visit. Even then, however, patients can leave feeling overwhelmed and confused.

There is also the problem of unrealistic expectations. We often seek health care assuming that all questions can be answered and all infections can be cured. But in reality medical professionals are not all-knowing or all-powerful, and herpes may force the issue. Faced with questions like "Where did I get this?" the healthcare provider may well have to say, "I don't know." Rightly or wrongly, this can lead to feelings of frustration and helplessness in the patient. And when it comes to the sexual or emotional impact of the diagnosis, providers may lack both the time and the specific training required.

Whatever the specifics of your situation, it's important to try to keep the lines of communication open. Patients should have a way to get answers, to get treatment if they need it, and to get advice on something that can affect their intimate relationships. If you feel you need some more time, you might try to schedule a follow-up visit to discuss your questions.

We know from interviews and from surveys that significant numbers of people with herpes voice complaints about their first visit and about the healthcare provider who first diagnosed them. In ASHA's 1991 survey, more than half rate this provider as "poor" or "fair" when asked specifically about the provider's performance in answering questions, giving treatment information, offering emotional support, and discussing a patient's sex life.

Worse still, a small number of patients report that their providers make them feel ashamed about having herpes and make remarks that assess blame—for example, comments like, "You now have to pay the consequences for what you've done." Another frequent complaint is that providers overlook the importance of leaving patients with a sense of hope or empowerment. Instead they may seem to be saying, "There is not much that can be done." Either kind of experience can have the effect of closing the door on further discussion of herpes. It can keep patients from asking the questions they need answered, getting treatment for current or future outbreaks, and getting advice they may want on a fairly intimate matter. It sets a negative tone that is hard to change.

Even if nothing especially awkward occurred during a first visit, herpes can have a chilling effect on open communication. Herpes may be difficult to talk about when we're first diagnosed—even with a medical professional. And this can pose a barrier to seeking further medical help, making one reluctant to ask certain questions or request follow-up consultations. Unfortunately, this cuts the patient off from a critical resource.

Among the benefits of professional medical care:

CORRECT DIAGNOSIS: People who try to diagnose themselves often regret it later. For example, a recent study has shown that 20% of patients seeking clinical care for genital symptoms were given a false positive diagnosis of genital herpes—that is, they were told they had herpes when they really didn't. Underdiagnosis of herpes is also a common problem. A confirming laboratory test can make all the difference, and it can be useful information to have for your medical records. In particular, knowing whether you have HSV-1 or HSV-2 may be helpful in predicting the course of the infection and in protecting partners. (For more on diagnostic tests, see Chapter 16.)

ACCESS TO ACUTE CARE: Patients with a first-episode infection are often sick for a couple of weeks or more and benefit from medication. The most effective medications are available only by prescription.

TREATMENT FOR RECCURENT GENITAL HERPES: For a variety of reasons, patients may wish to use medication for recurrent herpes. As we explain in Chapter 9, prescription medications may help to alleviate symptoms or dramatically reduce recurrence rates.

PREGNANCY: Women who have a history of genital herpes often need some advice about how to manage herpes if they choose to become pregnant. This advice relates not only to treatment but to the precautions that should be taken to avoid passing herpes to a newborn at delivery and immediately after. Management of herpes in pregnancy also is an issue for men with HSV whose partners are pregnant and have no history of herpes. (See Chapter 14.)

WHATEVER THE SPECIFICS of your situation, it's important to try to keep the lines of communication open. Patients should have a way to get answers, to get treatment if they need it, and to get advice on something that can affect their intimate relationships. It's important to remind yourself that strained or awkward relationships between the patient and the healthcare provider often can be repaired. If you feel you need some more time, you might try to schedule a follow-up visit to discuss your questions. However, if you are convinced you will not be comfortable seeking care for herpes with your current provider, there is always the option of looking for a "second opinion".

If you do feel it's time to look elsewhere for medical care, physicians with specialty training in gynecology, urology, dermatology, and infectious diseases may have more experience or technical training on herpes. On the other hand, it may be most important for you to have a clinician who will make you feel comfortable asking questions or who will be supportive emotionally, in which case a family practitioner or primary care provider may be the perfect choice. Much depends on the individuals involved.

You may be able to get a list of referrals from your local medical society or from a local herpes support group. If you have a university medical center or teaching hospital nearby, you can also reach the department dealing with infectious diseases and ask for a herpesvirus or STI specialist.

Another problem cited by people with herpes is a lack of continuity in care in today's large group practices and health maintenance organizations. You may work through the awkwardness of a first visit for genital herpes and get to feeling comfortable with one doctor or nurse practitioner, only to find that he or she isn't available the next time you need help. Do you make an appointment with someone else at the practice? Do you have to go through the hassle of discussing herpes again, your sex life again? Many people find this difficult. It's important to remember, though, that your health shouldn't take a back seat on account of shyness. Herpes may well prompt legitimate health questions and concerns from time to time. You should feel entitled to raise them. People who take charge and get the answers they want seldom look back and regret it.

WHAT YOU CAN DO

• Inform yourself about herpes and make a list of the questions and concerns you need to raise with a healthcare professional. Many people find it's a good idea to bring a written list when you have the medical consultation.

• It may take persistence to get the answers you need, but don't be afraid to ask your provider for help. Knowledge and emotional support are tools that can help put you back in control. If you have trouble broaching the subject, you might take a few minutes to ponder and rehearse a script. You might say, for example, "I feel awkward bringing this up, but I've had a history of genital herpes and there are some things that I've been wanting to get advice on." If the questions involve your partner, you might arrange to bring him or her along when you see your healthcare provider

• Ask the provider to explain your treatment options. Even if you decide not to use medications, knowledge is power. Don't let yourself feel cut off from treatment just because your provider isn't forthcoming about the options. As explained in Chapter 19, health insurance and managed care routinely cover antiviral medication for herpes. With the increased competition among chain and online pharmacies and with generic acyclovir available, cost may not be a barrier.

• If what you need is primarily emotional support, be realistic about what your medical professional can offer. Depending upon your personal situation, you may be best served by seeking out a friend or counselor or looking to other resources, such as the National Herpes Hotline or a local herpes support group. There is a list of Resources at the end of this book.

For some, these suggestions may beg the comment "easier said than done." Establishing good communication about herpes often takes a dose of hard work for both the patient and provider. Most experts stress three general points above all: Inform yourself; communicate your concerns and questions to your healthcare provider in an organized way; and don't be afraid to seek a second opinion if you're unsatisfied. The work might be hard, but it's a prescription you can write yourself.

9

TREATMENT OPTIONS

"My outbreaks were frequent and troublesome," writes Teri. "It wasn't so much because of the sores, which cleared up quickly, but because of symptoms like headache, tiredness, and muscle aches. It was like having the flu about once a month.

"I finally went to my gynecologist and started a course of drug therapy that has changed my life. I take medication every day, and now I'm symptom-free, in spite of a very stressful, demanding job and an active life.

"So far, so good, I guess. But I wonder how long it's safe to continue with this medication over the long term? And I wonder if there is a cure on the horizon."

The most common approach to treatment of genital herpes is the use of prescription antiviral drugs that are taken orally (by mouth). In this chapter, we will introduce the three leading antiviral medications. All three of these antivirals have been shown to be safe and effective based on overall clinical experience that ranges from 10 years of clinical studies to more than two decades. Each of these drugs helps to speed the healing of symptoms. In some cases, when taken daily, these drugs stop outbreaks altogether for long periods of time.

Equally important, one of the leading antivirals has been proven to significantly reduce the risk of spreading herpes to a partner.

As helpful as these drugs are, it's important to stress that today's antivirals do not cure herpes. They can't eliminate the herpes virus the way a specific antibiotic can knock out a specific kind of bacteria. Once a person is infected, HSV establishes latency and persists in the nerve ganglia. Today's drugs cannot prevent latency, but rather attack HSV and curb its spread at times when it becomes active and produces viral shedding.

While researchers continue to look for new, more effective treatments, the following three antiviral drugs approved by the U.S. Food and Drug Administration (FDA) comprise today's best treatment options based on clinical efficacy data. We will briefly describe the difference between these drugs first, and then explain the ways that they can be used later in the chapter.

ACYCLOVIR— The first antiviral to reach the market was acyclovir, sold under the brand name Zovirax® beginning in 1982 and available as an oral medication since 1985. Acyclovir is now a generic drug. It's truly a remarkable drug—one of the first to be effective against a virus without being toxic to normal cells. The scientist who led its development, Gertrude Elion, received a Nobel prize for her research.

Acyclovir works by attacking HSV's ability to reproduce. Like other viruses, HSV can move from cell to cell in its active phase, colonizing the cells as it goes and using them to create more virus. At the molecular level, the key to this process is the virus' genetic assembly instructions, or DNA (deoxyribonucleic acid). Acyclovir substitutes itself for one of the building blocks of the viral DNA and fools the virus into accepting an impostor. Once acyclovir has slipped into the machinery of the virus, the DNA chain stops.

For the patient taking the medication, this translates into a win over HSV, as viral shedding is brought to a standstill and symptoms go away. HSV, meanwhile, still has its safe haven—its base camp—in the nerve roots. In practical terms, a patient with a nasty first episode might normally have to wait three weeks before the skin lesions are healed and things have returned to normal. With acyclovir treatment, the length of the outbreak will be cut significantly.

In addition to acyclovir, people with herpes have a choice between two newer antivirals. Both are prodrugs, which means they have a kind of two-staged delivery. In stage one, you take the prodrug, which is then easily absorbed into the body. In stage two, the prodrug is converted by the body into the active medication.

VALACYCLOVIR — Valacyclovir (brand name Valtrex®) is currently marketed by GlaxoSmithKline. Valacyclovir is the prodrug of acyclovir, converting to acyclovir after ingestion. This process has the advantage of getting higher levels of acyclovir into the body. Most people absorb only 15% to 20% of acyclovir when they take it in conventional form, but taking the prodrug can boost absorption to the 50% to 80% range. In practical terms, valacyclovir has a couple of major advantages: One is less frequent dosing. The other is the capability to lower the risk of transmission from a person with genital herpes to a person who is not infected. We will discuss this in more detail later in this chapter.

FAMCICLOVIR — Famciclovir (brand name Famvir®), marketed by Novartis, is the prodrug of penciclovir. Famciclovir is more readily taken up by the body than penciclovir. It converts to penciclovir in the body, resulting in higher concentrations of the active drug than can be obtained with the oral administration. Like acyclovir, penciclovir works by fighting viral DNA. And like valacyclovir, famciclovir can be taken less often than acyclovir. A potential advantage of this drug is that a single-day regimen of famciclovir, when taken at first sign of an outbreak, is quite effective in controlling or preventing symptoms.

If your experience of genital herpes began with a marked first episode, you probably were given a prescription for one of these drugs. Given the large amounts of HSV present in first episodes, and given the immune system's lack of experience in fighting the virus, medication can have dramatic results.

Taken for seven to ten days, antiviral medication can shorten the duration of herpes symptoms (itching and pain, for instance) by 40% to 50%. It can reduce the length of time during which a first-episode patient is shedding virus—by 70% to 80%. And overall, it can mean a 30% to 40% decrease in the total time it takes for skin to heal. Not everyone has a painful first episode, but if you're suffering through one, these statistics may spell welcome relief. Dosages recommended for a first episode of genital herpes are given in Table 1, below.

TABLE 1. Recommended oral antiviral regimens for first episodes of genital herpes

NAME	BRAND	REGIMEN
Acyclovir	(generic)	400 mg, 3 times daily for 7-10 days
Acyclovir	(generic)	200 mg, 5 times daily for 7-10 days
Famciclovir	Famvir®	250 mg, 3 times daily for 7-10 days
Valacyclovir	Valtrex®	1000 mg, 2 times daily for 7-10 days

Does antiviral therapy work against recurrent genital herpes, too? It can, and here patients face a choice between two kinds of treatment. The first, called *episodic therapy*, means using medication to halt or shorten an outbreak once it has started. The second option, called *suppressive therapy,* means taking medicine every day in the hope that it will short-circuit reactivations of HSV, prevent outbreaks from occurring, and also help prevent transmission to a sexual partner.

EPISODIC THERAPY

One approach to using antiviral therapy is to treat an outbreak as it's unfolding. This type of treatment is called *episodic* therapy because one treats the individual episode and then stops taking medication until the next outbreak. With this approach, a patient begins taking medication at the first sign of recurrence.

First off, it's important to emphasize that antiviral therapy used for recurrent genital herpes gives less dramatic results than it does in first episodes. This is partly explained by the fact that the immune system is doing a lot of the work already. That's why recurrent outbreaks are usually much shorter than first episodes, anyway. In fact, the immune response is so effective that most of the viral replication during a recurrent episode occurs only during the first 48 hours.

Given the insight that most of the action takes place in the first two days of a recurrence, researchers have altered their approach to treating outbreaks. In the early days of acyclovir, one would typically take several doses per day for five days to treat a recurrence. Today, however, several new regimens have been tested that are shorter than the standard five-day course but utilize larger doses. Patients can take one-day, two-day, or three-day courses of treatment. The recommended antiviral dosages for episodic therapy of recurrent genital herpes are shown in Table 2 on the next page.

The results of episodic therapy vary quite a bit from person to person, but large controlled trials suggest the time to healing is gen-

TABLE 2. Recommended oral antiviral regimens for episodic therapy of recurrent genital herpes

NAME	BRAND	REGIMEN
Acyclovir	(generic)	400 mg, 3 times daily for 5 days
Acyclovir	(generic	800 mg, 2 times daily for 5 days
Acyclovir	(generic)	800 mg, 3 times daily for 2 days
Famciclovir	Famvir®	125 mg, 2 times daily for 5 days
Famciclovir	Famvir®	1000 mg, 2 times daily for 1 day
Valacyclovir	Valtrex®	500 mg, 2 times daily for 3 days
Valacyclovir	Valtrex®	1000 mg, 1 time daily for 5 days

erally reduced by an average of one to two days. The three drugs have not been compared head-to-head but all have roughly similar performance. Viral shedding may be reduced by half. Duration of symptoms (pain, tenderness, itching, tingling) may be reduced by 15% to 25%. And, if taken at the first sign of prodrome, episodic therapy can prevent an outbreak from occurring—aborting lesions, as the literature says—about 20% of the time with any of the antiviral drugs.

Regardless of which antiviral one is using, episodic therapy has its best results when medication is begun at the first sign of prodrome. If recurrent lesions are already present, therapy usually offers little benefit. For this reason, those taking episodic therapy should keep a supply of medication on hand so that they can start treatment when they first notice prodromal symptoms. The time required to involve a healthcare provider in this decision and obtain medication causes a significant delay in the start of treatment and is impractical. Most healthcare providers are already well aware of the advantages of giving their patients refillable prescriptions and will suggest this approach.

Overall, while clinical research has made headway in providing better options for treating outbreaks, many people feel the additional gains from episodic therapy are limited. For others, however, medication offers a useful way to manage outbreaks. This is especially true for those whose outbreaks tend to last more than a week.

SUPPRESSIVE THERAPY

While episodic therapy is a popular choice, people with herpes also have a second option called *suppressive therapy*. With this approach, one takes a smaller dose of antivirals every day in order to hold HSV in check and eliminate or "suppress" outbreaks. This obviously means paying more attention to a medication schedule but has a number of potential benefits worth considering: Suppressive therapy reduces the number of outbreaks by an average of 80% among people with frequent recurrences. For some, it can prevent outbreaks altogether for long periods. And it also has the potential to reduce the risk of HSV transmission to sexual partners.

As in the case of Teri, at the start of this chapter, many people find that suppressive antiviral treatment radically changes their experience of herpes, especially if they have frequent outbreaks. A long-term study has enrolled people who had frequent recurrences, put them on an acyclovir dose of 400 mg twice daily, and carefully tracked the results. In publishing the five-year data, researchers reported that nearly all patients on suppressive therapy had a dramatic reduction in the number of their outbreaks, beginning in the first year. They also found that people on this regimen experienced fewer and fewer recurrences, so that after one year, more than half of patients on suppressive therapy were completely free of outbreaks.

Famciclovir and valacyclovir, both approved in 1995, give similarly dramatic reductions in the number of outbreaks for most people.

It should also be noted that valacyclovir has the potential advantage of a once-daily regimen. For persons with fewer than 10 outbreaks per year, the approved suppressive dose of valacyclovir is 500 mg once daily. For those with 10 or more outbreaks per year the approved dose is 1 gram per day. All the recommended antiviral dosages for the suppression of recurrent genital herpes are shown in Table 3 below.

TABLE 3. Recommended oral antiviral regimens for suppression of recurrent genital herpes

NAME	BRAND	REGIMEN
Acyclovir	(generic)	400 mg, 2 times daily
Famciclovir	Famvir®	250 mg, 2 times daily
Valacyclovir	Valtrex®	500 mg, once daily (for people with fewer than 10 outbreaks per year)
Valacyclovir	Valtrex®	1000 mg, once daily

Preventing Viral Shedding and Transmission

It has been established for more than a decade that a daily regimen of any of these three antivirals dramatically reduces asymptomatic shedding. Clinical trials with acyclovir, famciclovir, and valacyclovir produced a reduction in viral shedding of anywhere from 80 to 94%. This was impressive, and raised the question of whether this effect on shedding would translate to lowering the risk of transmission between sexual partners.

The answer came in 2002, when researchers wrapped up a multinational study that examined the impact of daily suppressive therapy in monogamous "discordant" couples—1,484 heterosexual monogamous couples in which one partner had HSV-2 and the other did not. Over the course of 8 months, the couples were counseled on safer-sex practices and encouraged to use condoms during all sexual contacts. The partner with genital herpes was then given either a placebo (sugar pill) or put on a regimen of 500 mg of valacyclovir daily. The result? Those using valacyclovir cut the risk of transmission by 48%. In considering the merits of this data, the FDA approved valacyclovir's indication for reducing risk of heterosexual transmission for all persons with healthy immune systems. Though the initial study focused on monogamous couples where one person had a known history of herpes, the Centers for Disease Control and Prevention (CDC) state that suppressive valacyclovir probably reduces risk of transmission for persons who have multiple partners (including men who have sex with men) and those who are HSV-positive but have no history of symptoms.

While daily suppressive therapy with valacyclovir does not eliminate risk of transmission entirely, the fact that antivirals are in the prevention arsenal is a major gain for people who have genital HSV-2. Concern about protecting partners has always been a primary focus of people with herpes. Establishing that antiviral medication reduces risk of transmission of a viral infection is one of the major research gains of the past 20 years in the field.

Suppressive Treatment, Quality of Life, and Adjustment

We have already discussed the major potential benefits of preventing outbreaks and protecting sexual partners, but it's also worth mentioning that suppressive antiviral therapy has been studied for its potential benefits in improving patients' psychological and social adjustment. One multinational study found that suppressive therapy was correlated with statistically significant improvement in quality of life after 6 and 12 months of treatment.

Among healthcare professionals, the standard approach has

been to watch and wait as a newly diagnosed patient establishes a pattern of recurrences and then prescribe accordingly. When it was first approved for clinical use, suppressive therapy was most often prescribed for patients with frequent or troublesome recurrences. The idea was to wait and see how many recurrences a patient would have over the first year or two and then make a decision about using daily therapy.

Twenty years of research and clinical experience, however, now suggest a rationale for using suppressive therapy earlier in the course of patient management. Studies are now being done to evaluate the idea of routinely treating HSV-2 patients with suppressive therapy in the first six months following diagnosis. Theoretically, this approach delivers several benefits: First, it helps to control HSV reactivation—both outbreaks and asymptomatic shedding—during the year when patients generally experience the greatest number of reactivations. Second, it would help to lower the risk of transmission during the period when HSV is most likely transmitted. And third, it seems reasonable to believe that suppressive therapy might well help patients with any emotional adjustment that they need to make in the early months, when they are most likely to be distressed by a genital herpes diagnosis.

Dosing and Duration of Therapy

While suppressive therapy can be remarkably successful, it's important to note that some individuals simply do not respond well to a particular antiviral medication. In some cases, an increased dose is required to suppress HSV or a different medication is worth trying. For example, those who do not respond well to acyclovir may need as much as 800 mg. twice daily or may do better on one of the prodrugs. In a smaller number of cases, antivirals simply are not effective, suggesting the need for a different approach. Various regimens have been studied, and from the published research it seems that in general the effectiveness of suppressive therapy increases with the frequency of dosing. If you're wanting to alter the recommended suppressive therapy regimen, it's a good idea to discuss the issue with your medical professional.

Those on suppressive therapy may wish to stay on the drug indefinitely, and in the case of acyclovir, the safety of continuous therapy is established for up to 9 years. But many experts in the field suggest patients should talk with their healthcare providers from time to time about whether they continue to need suppressive treatment, possibly checking in after 12 consecutive months for what amounts to a reality check. Sometimes they won't have any outbreaks even without the drug, probably because of HSV's tendency to become less active after a number of years. Some people also find that their recurrences are less bothersome, so that they no longer want to take daily medication. The problem is that you have no way of knowing unless treatment is stopped for a while. For patients who continue to have a need for therapy, prescriptions can be renewed.

It's important to mention that patients discontinuing suppressive therapy should not be surprised to see a resumption of symptomatic recurrences in the short run. In a follow-up report on the patients in a long-term acyclovir study, researchers recorded the experiences of 239 patients who had stopped acyclovir suppressive therapy after 6 years of successful suppression. Among this group, 86% had at least one recurrence within a median of 68 days of stopping suppressive therapy and 75% had at least two recurrences within a median of 180 days after stopping suppressive therapy.

SAFETY CONCERNS

Over the years, many people with herpes have written ASHA with questions about the long-term safety of antiviral medication, particularly as used in suppressive therapy. Do these drugs have any toxic effects? Is suppressive therapy likely to give rise to drug-resistant strains of the virus or to weaken the body's natural immune response?

Suppressive therapy with acyclovir has been studied in thousands of patients over the past 15 years, and so far it appears to be very safe. In large trials, a small number of patients report side effects such as headaches, nausea, or diarrhea, but overall these complaints are rare. Researchers also have run laboratory tests to check for systemic effects of the drug on liver function, white blood cell count, and various other indexes of good health. So far, there is no evidence acyclovir causes harm to any internal organs. Thus far the safety data on the newer drugs are comparable to those for acyclovir, but they have not been used in people for as long as acyclovir.

The issue of resistant strains is more complicated. Within the universe of HSV-2, there are many different *strains* of the virus. For the most part, the differences among them are relevant only to molecular biologists. A small number of strains, however, are less sensitive to the effects of the three antiviral drugs that we have discussed in this chapter. One reason for this lack of sensitivity is that some strains actually lack the enzyme (thymidine kinase) that triggers these drugs and enables them to thwart the virus in its effort to spread. These strains are rare, can arise spontaneously, and typically have only a small proportion of viral particles that lack thymidine kinase. For this reason, the immune system generally can control these viral strains in healthy people.

In patients who have weakened immune systems, however, these strains can cause serious illness, because the immune system can't do its customary work in suppressing herpes, and resistant strains can replicate without much interference. People with AIDS, for example, may have severe herpes outbreaks that do not heal with conventional antiviral medication. Alternate treatments are now being used for these patients.

Is the problem of drug resistance likely to increase over time, as more and more people take antivirals? It appears unlikely. Researchers have actually checked samples of HSV taken before the development of acyclovir, and they find a small percentage of viral strains that are naturally less sensitive to the drug. Surprisingly, this number has not changed, despite wide use of the drug. However, in immune-deficient patients, all strains of the virus grow better, and treatment with antivirals may allow resistant strains to survive and prosper. Some scientists believe that HSV does mutate over time, and it's possible that acyclovir—or any antiviral drug—will exert pressure for certain strains of the virus to survive better than others.

For now, the experts say, the odds of developing acyclovir-resistant herpes are extremely low in people with normal immune systems. Researchers have looked for resistant strains in people taking acyclovir daily for up to 6 years and found no evidence of increasing resistance. A survey of herpes patients in northwest England reported that resistant strains of the herpes virus were found with equal prevalence (0.1% to 0.6% of virus samples tested) among immuno-competent patients who had been treated with acyclovir and among those who had not received acyclovir. The issue of drug-resistance in those with weakened immunity, by contrast, is of more immediate concern, and immunocompromised patients with herpes should be monitored closely if they're taking antiviral medication.

HIV AND IMMUNE-SUPPRESSED PATIENTS

First, a person who has HIV infection should not jump to the conclusion that the frontline antiviral treatments will be ineffective for them. In fact, the three established HSV treatments play an important role in helping HIV-positive persons manage their health.

To begin with, because of immune suppression, persons with HIV have more frequent HSV reactivations—both in the form of lesion-causing recurrences and asymptomatic shedding. Outbreaks can be severe, and even with treatment lesions may require longer healing times. Equally important, HSV-2 and HIV interact in ways that create two kinds of risks. First, the presence of both herpes-infected and HIV-infected cells can potentially increase the HIV viral load, which poses its own health risk. Second, this interaction between the viruses increases the likelihood of HIV transmission and of HSV transmission.

As a result, the dosing regimens for persons with HIV are more stringent. With episodic treatment, short-course regimens should not be used; each of the antivirals should be continued for five to 10 days, and higher doses are often needed. The recommended regimens for episodic treatment of recurrent genital herpes in persons with HIV are shown in Table 4 below.

TABLE 4. Recommended oral antiviral regimens for episodic treatment of recurrent genital herpes in persons infected with HIV

NAME	BRAND	REGIMEN
Acyclovir	(generic)	400 mg, 3 times daily for 5-10 days
Famciclovir	Famvir®	500 mg, 2 times daily for 5-10 days
Valacyclovir	Valtrex®	1000 mg, 2 times daily for 5-10 days

Because of the interaction between HSV-2 and HIV, many

experts today recommend that patients who test positive for both viral infections stay on suppressive therapy. The goal is to prevent troublesome HSV symptoms and simultaneously help to control HIV viral load. In fact, suppressive therapy for HSV is routinely used to control all forms of HSV reactivation (including oral-facial HSV) in a range of immune-suppressed patients, such as persons receiving chemotherapy or undergoing a transplant. The recommended regimens for suppressive treatment of recurrent herpes in HIV-positive persons are shown in Table 5 below.

TABLE 5. Recommended oral antiviral regimens for suppression of recurrent genital herpes in persons infected with HIV

NAME	BRAND	REGIMEN
Acyclovir	(generic)	400-800 mg, 2-3 times daily
Famciclovir	Famvir®	500 mg, 2 times daily
Valacyclovir	Valtrex®	500 mg, 2 times daily

There are cases when the frontline treatments do not work adequately. In some cases, foscarnet is used as an alternative therapy for immunocompromised patients who don't respond well to acyclovir. Like acyclovir, foscarnet blocks viral replication, but it does so by working directly against a viral enzyme called *polymerase*. It isn't readily absorbed through the stomach, and must be administered intravenously. Other second-line treatment options include topical cidofovir gel, which is applied to the recurrent lesions once daily for five days, and a topical agent called imiquimod, which belongs to the class of drugs called immune modulators. Administered topically, imiquimod is designed to stimulate a strong local immune response and does work in some HIV patients. The antiviral compound, trifluridine, is also sometimes used topically to treat herpes infections that do not respond to other therapies.

COMPARISON SHOPPING

How does one evaluate the available treatments? Let's consider four major aspects: Effectiveness, safety, convenience, and cost.

In terms of effectiveness for people with established HSV infection, clinical studies generally have found few significant differences between acyclovir, famciclovir, and valacyclovir. All three appear to work for the vast majority of patients as a suppressive therapy and to have modest but reliable benefit as episodic therapy. While there are few head-to-head studies comparing these drugs, a paper published in 2006 showed that valacyclovir had a slight edge over famciclovir as a suppressive treatment. Study subjects taking daily valacyclovir had less confirmed viral shedding during the 10-week study period, and were able to remain free of viral shedding for a longer period of time than those in the famciclovir group.

Reducing the risk of transmission, of course, is the other key efficacy issue. Valacyclovir has produced solid clinical data supporting the drug's ability to partially reduce the risk of transmission and is approved for this indication by the FDA. How other drugs would compare for that indication is not known.

As for safety, it can be argued that acyclovir has an edge by virtue of its long track record, with no evidence of toxicity even in those who have been taking daily medication for years. However, the newer drugs also appear to be very safe and have few side effects. Valacyclovir, which uses acyclovir as its active ingredient, has shown a similar safety profile so far, as has famciclovir. Perhaps, with time, the prodrugs will match acyclovir's record fully.

Convenience probably offers a slight edge to the newer drugs.

Famciclovir has an edge in episodic therapy with its FDA-approved one-day regimen. Valacyclovir and acyclovir, by contrast, must be taken two or three times a daily at a minimum (see Tables 2 and 3). For suppression, valacyclovir achieves good results in most people with a once-daily dose, something that neither of its competitors has been able to match. While this is significant to some patients, it should also be noted the valacyclovir transmission study used a once daily dose that reduced risk by 48%, which suggests that some break-through viral shedding was occurring with this regimen. A higher dose or more frequent dose (twice daily) may produce better results.

Cost, of course, is the other critical issue. Here there is actually good news. In the decade since this book was first published, the availability of generic acyclovir, price competition among national chain pharmacies, the start or presence of online pharmacies, and increased use of prescription drug cards by insurers have combined to make antiviral medication more affordable and easier to obtain. Nonetheless, in today's healthcare arena, a given patient's treatment options are highly dependent on the insurer's regulations and poli-cies. One type of health plan might place generic acyclovir in its for-mulary; another might go with one of the prodrugs.

If, on the other hand, you will be paying out of pocket for a long-term course of therapy, it would be smart to research the cost of each of the three drugs to determine which is the best value in your particular market. For suppressive therapy, for example, what is the cost to you of twice daily generic acyclovir versus once daily valacy-clovir? How does your local pharmacy's price compare with those of the national chains? And what are the online pharmacies charging? There is an enormous range in prices for six months of suppressive therapy though on-line vendors. As of this writing, prices are as low as $150 for a year of suppressive therapy with generic acyclovir supplied by an on-line pharmacy, and discounts could be found for the prodrugs as well. Take time to research your best options.

In the end, all three antivirals can be considered safe and effective, but the hit to one's pocketbook may vary dramatically according to health insurance, geography, and the pricing structure at your preferred pharmacy.

CONSIDERING TREATMENT FOR YOURSELF

In today's healthcare environment, a person diagnosed with first episode genital herpes is most likely to receive a course of antiviral therapy to hasten healing of these initial symptoms. But what then? Is it best to keep a supply of an antiviral on hand in case of recurrences? Is daily suppressive therapy something to consider? Who makes the call?

There are no simple guidelines to offer, because every patient's circumstances are different. The patient's medical history, the impact of herpes on the patient's life, and the patient's and healthcare provider's views regarding treatment—all come into play.

Ideally, however, one constant here will be a dialogue between patient and provider concerning the impact of herpes and the therapeutic options. Here are some issues to weigh:

• What is the infecting type: HSV-1 or HSV-2? As we explained earlier, HSV-1 is unlikely to cause a pattern of frequent recurrences and appears less likely to cause asymptomatic shedding as well. With HSV-2, on the other hand, symptomatic recurrences are virtually a sure thing, and rates of asymptomatic shedding are higher.

• Are you and your partner very concerned about the risk of transmission? For people who want to do everything they can to reduce this risk, suppressive therapy is a logical addition to other prevention strategies.

• Are you already experiencing a pattern of frequent or painful outbreaks? A pattern of recurrent outbreaks six or more times a year leads some patients to use suppressive antiviral therapy, especially if the outbreaks are lengthy or painful. But the threshold is different for everyone. In any case, your doctor has no way to gauge this other than your honest assessment. Try to communicate this information.

• Is anxiety about recurrences substantially affecting your life? Does recurrent herpes take an emotional toll on you? Even people who get just a handful of outbreaks each year may feel the need for antiviral treatment if, for example, they are facing a time of stress during which herpes is the last thing they want to contend with. One example: Persons recently divorced or on their own after the breakup of a long-term relationship might suddenly feel anxiety about herpes and seek advice on treatment for the first time.

• Do your recurrences last a long time? The average duration of recurrences is about four to six days, and in these cases, episodic treatment may not bring a substantial improvement. Persons with longer recurrences might benefit significantly from episodic treatments. Those with frequent but brief recurrences might get more benefit from suppressive treatment.

• Are you pregnant, or trying to get pregnant? The medications mentioned here should not be used during pregnancy without consulting a specialist, though antivirals are indicated for specific situations that might arise during pregnancy. (See Chapter 14 for more on this.)

The most important piece of advice here is to focus on your needs and speak up for yourself in this decision-making process. All too often, patients receive a prescription for treatment of a first episode and then get little followup in the next few months. If a patient is somewhat embarrassed to bring up the subject, the result is that they have little or no chance to discuss the impact of herpes and the potential role of treatment. Don't let that happen.

10

TOPICAL TREATMENTS AND ALTERNATIVE APPROACHES

Chapter 9 covered the three antiviral drugs with a strong clinical track record for effectiveness and safety in treating genital herpes. To put this in some perspective, acyclovir, famciclovir, and valacyclovir are the only three drugs indicated for people with healthy immune systems in the current treatment guidelines for genital herpes from the U. S. Centers for Disease Control and Prevention (CDC). At the same time, it's clear that many people with HSV infections are interested in other approaches to treatment. In this chapter we will review what is known about some of these options, ranging from topical treatments to complementary and alternative therapies.

TOPICAL THERAPY

Because herpes was originally perceived as a skin condition, the idea of topical medication has always had some appeal. Over the past three decades a number of different compounds have been developed for topical application to herpes lesions, though it has proved difficult to make a drug that's absorbed through the skin well enough to provide substantial relief. Acyclovir was initially tested and approved as a topical ointment for genital herpes in 1982. Results with oral acyclovir were far superior, however, and since 1985 acyclovir cream has not been recommended for genital herpes. Although none of the topical therapies studied so far has been on par with oral therapy, the effort to develop more effective topicals continues.

ACYCLOVIR — Though they clearly do not pack the punch of the oral drug, acyclovir-based topical formulations are still available. Biovail Pharmaceuticals markets both a 5% acyclovir cream and 5% ointment under acyclovir's original brand name, Zovirax®. The cream has FDA approval for treatment of recurrent cold sores only—not genital herpes. The ointment has an indication for treatment of initial genital herpes episodes but not for recurrences. In 2006, the FDA warned Biovail that its promotional material tended to overstate the effectiveness of the ointment and to falsely imply it might have a role in controlling transmission. The FDA emphasized the ointment has no clinical benefit in treating or suppressing recurrent genital herpes.

PENCICLOVIR — Penciclovir, the active ingredient in famciclovir, is available as a topical cream and has been investigated for the treatment of oral and genital herpes. A 1% penciclovir cream known as Denavir® can be purchased over-the-counter for treatment of cold sores on the lips and face. This topical formulation shortens the duration of pain and healing time for cold sore patients when applied every two hours (during waking hours), and also appears to reduce viral shedding. The usefulness of this drug for genital herpes, however, remains questionable. A clinical trial comparing penciclovir cream and acyclovir cream for genital herpes found no clinically significant differences between the two drugs. However, a placebo group was not included in the trial, which makes evaluation difficult.

DOCOSANOL — In 2000, the FDA approved a new non-prescription cream medication for oral herpes called docosanol, marketed as Abreva®. Docosanol's mode of action is different from that of acyclovir or penciclovir; docosanol is thought to disrupt the process by which the herpes virus particle gains entry to the uninfected cell. One small placebo-controlled study (63 patients) of docosanol for recurrent cold sores found that early application, i.e., at first "tingling sensation" or at the first appearance of any redness, shortened healing time by approximately 3 days. This product has not been studied thoroughly for genital herpes and as such is not recommended by CDC or other policy-setting groups.

TOPICAL ANESTHETICS — Other topical drugs, while they make no claim to stop viral replication, may relieve symptoms in other ways. Topical lidocaine partially (and temporarily) numbs the nerve endings and is occasionally used to treat the pain of first episodes. However, it's not widely used for herpes, and people using it should be aware of the possibility of allergic reactions to this and similar drugs such as novocaine. The FDA has approved a patch version of topical lidocaine (Lidoderm®) for the symptomatic treatment of post-herpetic neuralgia, the very painful after-effect of the herpes zoster viral infection known as shingles. The usefulness of this patch for HSV-related neuralgia has not been studied. [A placebo-controlled study of 1.8% tetracaine cream for oral herpes reported a 30% reduction in healing time (about 2 days); however, here again there is a lack of published data on tetracaine for genital herpes.]

OVER-THE-COUNTER MEDICATIONS — People with herpes sometimes try over-the-counter products to relieve the symptoms of a flare-up. It's difficult to assess the value of these medications because they generally are not tested as rigorously as the prescription drugs discussed in this chapter and are not evaluated in the scientific literature. In some cases, neither are they labeled specifically for use in the treatment of genital herpes. They nonetheless attract attention through word-of-mouth, or because they claim to erase whatever kind of symptom is most distressing to the patient—itching, for example.

Unfortunately, topical creams may actually delay the healing of herpes outbreaks. In some cases, the creams contain alcohol compounds that might dry the skin to the point where it is easily chafed. Other topical treatments, such as Campho-Phenique®, may make patients feel better because the product contains phenol. Like xylocaine and lidocaine, phenol numbs the area locally, without treating the actual infection. Some people may find this useful. It's important to note, however, that products such as Campho-Phenique® or Blistex® do not actually work directly against the virus—they concentrate instead on the symptoms of viral attack.

Other topical medications—even prescription drugs—can have a downside when it comes to herpes. Some doctors use topical steroid creams to reduce inflammation and speed healing for a variety of skin problems. Unfortunately, steroids cause some immune impairment, and this may make a herpesvirus infection worse, decreasing the ability of the skin to heal on its own. Steroids are not effective for HSV, and they can prolong herpes outbreaks. Topical steroids such as hydrocortisone may increase the risk of yeast infection as well. (By the way, people taking steroids for other conditions, such as asthma, sometimes report that their herpes outbreaks are worse as a result.)

While the products mentioned here may have uses in some circumstances, oral antivirals have a superior clinical track record for safety and effectiveness. If you want more information about a prescription or over-the-counter product for treating symptoms of genital herpes, one option is to contact the Office of Consumer Affairs at the FDA. (See the Resource List on page 221.) They can discuss drugs that are labeled specifically for treatment of genital herpes. Another option is to contact the product's manufacturer.

COMPLEMENTARY AND ALTERNATIVE MEDICINES

Among those who find herpes troubling, some look for alternatives in managing the infection, often because of the expense or the inconvenience of prescription medications, or because they have philosophical objections to them. They look for other ways to take control. In several surveys over the past 15 years, results show that a significant percentage of people with herpes experiment with treatments or management strategies outside the traditional medical model, including dietary supplements and nutritional approaches. There are also advocates for hypnosis, homeopathy, acupuncture, naturopathy, chiropractic, psychotherapy, visualization, herbal remedies, traditional Chinese medicine, and more.

The list is long, and it changes each year. The movement toward alternative medicine, in fact, is a national trend of considerable scope. According to a survey published in 2004, more than 36% of Americans were using some form of complementary and alternative therapy. It's estimated that we spend $47 billion a year in the process. Partly as a result, the National Institutes of Health (NIH) has now set up a special branch, the National Center for Complementary and

Alternative Medicine (NCCAM), which funds rigorous studies of alternative approaches to treatment.

Unfortunately, until more of these studies on herpes-related treatments in alternative medicine are completed and published, it's difficult to evaluate the compounds in question, Most complementary and alternative medicines (CAM) are not scientifically tested and retested like prescription drugs, and in the vast majority of cases, there are no double-blind studies, so one can never be sure that the results have been free of bias. These therapies also lack an approval process that hinges on the performance of a given treatment in a large cross-section of people. In addition, with natural products such as echinacea and ginseng, we are faced with the issue that there can be multiple pharmacologically active constituents. There can also be great variability in the ingredients based on factors such as variations in plant parts used, local growing and processing techniques, extraction methods, and product formulations.

Although herpes has not yet figured largely in studies funded by NIH, in 2005 a group of researchers at the University of Texas (Galveston) reviewed the published literature on CAM treatments for genital HSV and listed 21 compounds that had been reviewed in at least one scientific journal. From these, in an article published in the journal *HERPES* in 2005, authors Michelle Perfect et al. provided a summary of six common CAM options that had shown some promise and had been tested in human trials: Echinacea, eleuthero, l-lysine, zinc, bee products, and aloe vera.

While most of these did not have compelling evidence behind them, three appeared worthy of serious follow up study to resolve questions. Bee products included honey and propolis, a sticky substance that bees produce from certain tree saps. Both are inexpensive and likely to prove safe, and both exhibited some effectiveness when administered topically. (The honey was used directly on lesions; the propolis was delivered in an ointment.) In addition, the common herbal remedy aloe vera was shown to be active against HSV in the laboratory and to accelerate healing by a modest amount in human subjects when used in a topical preparation.

The third product listed, L-lysine, is perhaps the most often-

COMPLEMENTARY AND ALTERNATIVE MEDICINE TREATMENTS USED FOR GENITAL HERPES

COMMON NAMES	METHOD OF APPLICATION
ALGAE/SEAWEED	ORAL OR TOPICAL
ALOE VERA	TOPICAL
ASTRAGALUS	ORAL
BUTYLATED HYDROXYTOLUENE (BHT)	DIET OR ORAL
BEE PRODUCTS	TOPICAL
DRAGON'S BLOOD	ORAL OR TOPICAL
ECHINACEA	ORAL
EUCALYPTUS OIL	TOPICAL
ELEUTHERO/SIBERIAN GINSENG	ORAL
GARLIC	DIET, ORAL, OR TOPICAL
LIQUORICE	ORAL OR TOPICAL
LITHIUM	ORAL OR TOPICAL
L-LYSINE	DIET OR ORAL
LEMON BALM/MELISSA	ORAL OR TOPICAL
PEPPERMINT OIL	TOPICAL
PRUNELLA VULGARIS	TOPICAL
RESVERATROL	DIET OR TOPICAL
ST. JOHN'S WORT	ORAL OR TOPICAL
TEA TREE OIL	TOPICAL
VITAMINS	DIET, ORAL, OR TOPICAL
ZINC	DIET, ORAL, OR TOPICAL

Source: CAM and Genital Herpes. HERPES, 12:2 2005

tried approach and therefore worthy of additional discussion. One of the essential amino acids that the body uses to build proteins, L-lysine is a natural part of many foods we consume, such as meat, milk, and eggs. Beginning in the late 1970s, a small number of nutritional researchers began to claim that people who consumed abnormally large quantities of L-lysine on a daily basis had fewer herpes flare-ups and recovered from them more quickly. In one study, subjects took 3,000 mg of L-lysine every day to achieve these gains. Unfortunately, other studies reached contradictory findings, and it's difficult to interpret the results because the study populations, doses, and endpoints varied so widely. Some might say the jury is still out.

While CAM approaches such as L-lysine may be helpful with herpes symptoms, it's relevant to consider how well their effectiveness compares with generic acyclovir or other FDA-approved antiviral drugs. In the studies of bee products and aloe vera mentioned above, the products were seen to show promise if they performed better than acyclovir cream or improved healing times in patients with symptoms lasting 10 days to two weeks. Neither measure sets the bar very high when you compare these data to recent trials of the prescription episodic therapies recommended in the CDC's treatment guidelines for genital herpes. By the same token, there is also more safety data for the oral antivirals.

Additionally, the emphasis for many CAM treatments is on symptomatic relief—speeding the healing of lesions. Today, however, asymptomatic shedding and transmission are the central issues to many people with herpes, and we have little or no data on these more complex aspects of therapy and how CAM products perform.

It's also worth considering that some alternative therapies, even megadoses of vitamins, are quite costly. One would tend to think that prescription pharmaceutical products are always going to be the more costly choice. But when it comes to HSV, generic acyclovir significantly changes the playing field. Whatever the future benefits of CAM products might be, if you currently have frequent outbreaks, antiviral therapy may give you significantly more gain for your drugstore dollar than nutritional supplements or herbal remedies.

11

SORTING OUT THE EMOTIONAL ISSUES

"I've had herpes for a year now," says Ruth. "I was able to figure out the medical part of it pretty quickly—how to recognize symptoms and what treatment suited me. The hardest part was I was still single when I got it, so I had difficulty figuring out when and how to tell someone about herpes. But I've been lucky in love, I guess. I've found someone special. As far as adjusting to herpes, I'm 'over it,' as the saying goes."

"When I acquired herpes seven months ago," says Sean, "I was shattered. I remember sitting there in the dark listening to Pink Floyd's 'Comfortably Numb,' which is exactly what I was (thanks to the sedatives my doctor had given me)."

When we're first diagnosed with genital herpes, much of what we learn has to do with the physical impact of herpes. But it's well-accepted by now that for many people herpes also has emotional consequences. There are dozens of studies that have assessed the social and psychological effects of herpes. Especially in the first few weeks and months, herpes can affect self-image, make one feel isolated or embarrassed, and complicate relationships. For some of us, these issues can be just as troublesome—and sometimes much more so— than physical symptoms.

The good news is that these problems tend to fade away with time. In fact, some studies show that a few weeks or a few months can make a big difference in adjusting to herpes.

Your own response depends on the circumstances of your life. For some, the emotional impact of herpes may be minimal, even at the start. If, however, there are some tough personal issues raised by a recent herpes diagnosis, it can be very helpful to sort them out, analyze what's upsetting you, and think through some approaches to resolving them.

HERPES AND SELF-IMAGE

Many people describe herpes as shaking their self-confidence or making them think of themselves as less worthy. For example, a young woman who had acquired herpes as a teenager wrote: "I had times when I would feel very unattractive and feel like I was different from everyone my own age. The best way I can sum it up is that I felt 'dirty.'"

Why does herpes have the power to alter our self-image? In some ways this is truly a paradox. HSV is a common virus, and most adults already have HSV-1, the usual cause of cold sores. Most of us have had other herpesviruses as well. Examples include the viruses that cause chickenpox, mononucleosis, and the childhood infection roseola. In some ways, then, the anxiety we feel about HSV makes no sense.

Psychologists point out that numerous chronic health conditions adversely affect self-image or self-esteem, and this seems to be an issue with herpes. The lack of a cure and the prospect of recurrent symptoms are stressful thoughts for some as they think through what herpes will mean for their lives.

Too often we see health as an all-or-nothing proposition—we are either healthy or unhealthy, with no middle ground. And some people regard a chronic infection like herpes as the end of health. We become somehow imperfect.

In reality, however, health involves a process of growth and change. Everyone faces a host of physical challenges as inevitable as life itself. Whether it's a cold, the flu, allergies, an ear infection, or anything else, the task is to meet them head on and get past them. Herpes is no exception. In the end, we should consider ourselves healthy because we meet the challenges that life throws our way.

Herpes can also threaten our self-image in an area where many of us feel a bit vulnerable already: Our feelings of sexual desirability. Sociologist Sevgi Aral comments that people carry around with them a good deal of general anxiety about their attractiveness to a potential partner. Feelings of insecurity such as these are commonplace, and herpes adds a complication, another potential barrier to intimacy.

The impact of herpes on one's sex life might be challenging, but this too can be addressed—first, by learning to talk about it, and second, by making rational decisions about protecting a partner. Studies show that, with time, newly diagnosed persons usually overcome the distress they often feel about the effect of herpes on sexual relationships. We will discuss this further in Chapter 13.

SOCIAL STIGMA?

Closely connected to the issue of self-image is the matter of how we believe others see us. In many cases, the person with herpes will assume that society regards him or her as different in some substantial way. This, in essence, is the definition of social stigma. It's a feeling that one is *marked* by herpes—that it's more just than a medical condition.

Interestingly, though, sociologists who study this topic point out that people may assume that something carries social stigma when it doesn't, or may exaggerate the potential for stigma. A less-than-sensitive remark by a doctor, for example, can cast a long shadow psychologically. And herpes jokes of the type sometimes heard on late-night TV can touch a nerve for some. These may go unremarked by much of the listening audience. But for too many of those diagnosed with herpes every year, these jokes may feed self-doubt and reinforce feelings of isolation.

These kinds of remarks build a sort of mythology that can make it hard on people newly diagnosed with herpes, but the reaction you might get from real people in your life is most often quite different. Talking to a close friend about herpes may show you an entirely different reality. Lots of people know that herpes is a very common infection, and lots of people know someone who has herpes. In other words, you may see evidence of social stigma in various places, but you don't have to let it set the tone in your own life.

So why don't people talk about herpes more? As a society, we're still not comfortable with honest discussion about all aspects of sexuality. Today, we're surrounded by the imagery of sex in arts, entertainment, and advertising of products as diverse as soft drinks and automobiles. There are some signs as well that on a personal level we are becoming somewhat more open about sexuality—more likely to discuss topics such as sexual orientation and sexual function. All the same, these topics still are not the easiest to bring up in conversation.

A good example is the enormous amount of press and conversation triggered by the launch of Viagra® in 1998, including the television commercials featuring retired U.S. Senator Bob Dole. As a society we certainly talked about the issue of sexual dysfunction as we never had before, but we still had some discomfort and embarrassment with a subject that had long been kept out of public discourse. Hence the spate of jokes and editorial cartoons.

One form of progress on this front is the effort to make health-care providers more aware of how widespread herpes is. A major study published in 2003 by Douglas Fleming and colleagues recruited a random sample of patients from suburban primary care clinics and tested them for HSV-2. Of the 5,452 study subjects between the ages of 18 and 59, 25.5% tested positive for HSV-2. In publicizing these results, Fleming and his co-authors stressed that too often clinicians view herpes and other STIs as an issue only in "high-risk populations." In fact, as the study showed, even in affluent patients with access to care, the numbers are high—and clinicians should be better prepared to diagnose and treat HSV.

Certainly in the mass media, there has been some small headway in the discussion of herpes. Prime-time television advertising appears to have raised awareness, and surveys show that the public is much better educated about the subject today than ever before. Perhaps the day will come when even the idea of social stigma connected to herpes is a distant memory.

TALKING ABOUT HERPES

In the meantime, of course, it may be a bit awkward or embarrassing to discuss herpes with various people in your life, and many people worry for a while about the practical impact of herpes on important relationships. Do you dare tell people? Will discussing herpes damage a relationship you have now? Will a future romantic interest understand and accept the news?

These anxieties are natural, but it's important to overcome them. If you are withdrawing from friends or intimate relationships because of what you've internalized as social stigma, you run the risk of cutting yourself off from the support you need to keep everything in perspective. Studies have shown that social support is one of the most important factors in ensuring that herpes doesn't interfere with your life over the long haul.

Psychologist Cal VanderPlate, who has studied the behavioral effects of herpes, says that the key to keeping herpes in perspective is communication. People who can tell a partner or a friend about herpes often get emotional support from this person when they need it.

Talking about herpes, even with someone you love and trust, can be daunting at first. And herpes isn't likely to be something that you will choose to bring up with just anyone. In surveys, people most frequently report discussing herpes with their healthcare provider and with their spouse or partner, though not everyone does.

Perhaps the most pressing worry for those newly diagnosed with herpes is the reaction of a sexual partner. Feelings of suspicion or resentment can be a factor in some cases, as a couple tries to sort out the source of the herpes infection. On the other hand, if blame is not an issue, those who already have a steady partner potentially have a wonderful source of emotional support that can ease their adjustment.

People often say they especially fear telling a new partner or romantic interest because they're afraid of being rejected. They particularly worry about herpes being contagious, and about how the conversation is going to go when they have to talk about which precautions they might use. "I've had herpes for three months now, and I've been avoiding any sexual entanglements," writes Pat. "I'm not ready to tell anyone. I just don't think I'll be able to handle it if someone rejects me because of this." Experts say the best way to approach talking to a partner about herpes is to think through what you are going to say—perhaps even rehearse it—and then say it in a direct, honest, and upbeat way. (Telling a partner and thinking through the issue of prevention are explored in depth in the next two chapters.)

Support can come from a friend as well. In any case, the key is having someone to talk to, but this requires honesty and openness on the part of the person with herpes. Usually, says VanderPlate, acceptance and support are just around the corner, but we never know unless we take the risk. You may need a little time first, but opening up to a trusted friend may be exactly the boost you need to put things in perspective and get on with your life.

HERPES AND SEXUAL HEALTH

As we mentioned earlier, sexuality appears to be an area where most people experience insecurity from time to time, and having a chronic infection that is sexually transmitted can exacerbate these insecurities. In addition, there are practical issues. Having an infection that can reactivate and become contagious at unpredictable times does present some challenges. Herpes can interfere with sex when symptoms are present. And it can raise the issue of risk reduction measures between outbreaks, including daily antivirals, condom use, and other measures.

As with other aspects of the emotional and social adjustment, surveys show that some people find herpes affects their enjoyment of sex and their spontaneity. But here again, the negative effects are often short-term. After a period of adjustment, most people have sex just as often and enjoy it just as much as they did before.

Most people with herpes naturally do worry about transmitting herpes to a sexual partner, and having a sexual relationship does mean considering the risks: When is herpes active? What, precisely, are *my* symptoms? Is my partner at risk—or does he or she already have it? Do we need to use condoms or some other form of risk reduction?

There *are* things you can do to lower the risk of spreading herpes. Experts believe that simply knowing your symptoms and refraining from sexual contact during symptomatic times is an important precaution. Suppressive antiviral therapy with valacyclovir—meaning consistent daily doses—has a proven effect in lowering the risk. Use of condoms in between outbreaks also has significant value. All of these issues are covered in more detail in Chapter 13.

In addition to the sexual impact of herpes, people often wonder if the burden of having herpes—and possibly transmitting it—will become a serious problem over the long term. ASHA has interviewed many couples about this issue and found no indication that herpes has to stand in the way of successful, enduring relationships. One woman who doesn't have herpes wrote ASHA with the specific aim of making this very point. "Some people with herpes seem to give up on relationships," she commented, "so I wanted to share my story. My husband is the love of my life. We've been married almost 10 years, and herpes hasn't spoiled our relationship in any way. Like almost everyone else, we've had our problems, but herpes isn't one of them."

Asked about herpes and long-term relationships, psychologists concur that it's basically a non-issue in a healthy relationship. As long as two people are honest with each other at the start, as long as they can talk about herpes and make choices about it, the infection itself becomes just one more practical matter to deal with—usually a small one.

EMOTIONS AND ADJUSTMENT

Issues of self-esteem, fear of rejection, and anxieties about one's sex life are common among those newly diagnosed, and herpes can have other emotional consequences as well. A number of studies have documented anxiety in a percentage of newly diagnosed patients as well as feelings of depression or other signs of psychological distress. As we have mentioned earlier, however, even those who have initially had a difficult time with herpes often go through a process of adjustment after which they are functioning—and feeling—much the way they did before their diagnosis.

In raising the possibility of consequences such as depression, our purpose is not to characterize herpes as psychologically crippling. Rather it's to allow for the possibility that a newly diagnosed patient may have a wide variety of emotional responses. Though these responses are usually short term, a person who is suffering greatly may benefit from taking aggressive steps to treat herpes and to seek help from a professional counselor who can help sort through the issues that the diagnosis has raised.

MOVING FORWARD

If having herpes is causing you a lot of emotional stress, here are some points to keep in mind:

- Realize that it's normal to be stressed emotionally by herpes, especially at first. Give yourself some time to adjust, and remember that the emotional issues will get easier.

• Keep in mind that genital herpes is somewhat like other infections you may have had in the past. You are capable of managing it.

• If you're feeling isolated, you may need to find someone to talk to. Perhaps you might pick one close friend and tell her or him about it. You can ask that the conversation be kept in absolute confidence.

• Do not make the assumption that having herpes will prevent you from being romantically involved or having successful long-term relationships. There are millions of couples in which one or both partners have this infection. Relationships stand or fall on far more important issues.

12

TELLING A PARTNER

Carl, now 38, remembers the first few conversations he had about herpes. "When I got the diagnosis, I was able to make phone calls to the two people I'd been intimate with and ask if either of them had any idea they had herpes. I wasn't so much angry at that point as worried and wanting to be, I guess, responsible about it. So it wasn't that hard to make the calls. But later, when it came time to tell someone new, I lost my nerve at first. I really couldn't stand the idea that it might make someone feel differently about me."

The prospect of telling another person you have herpes can make you anxious, especially when you're getting ready to tell someone with whom you'd like to be sexually intimate. How will this person react? Will they be difficult? Accept that herpes doesn't have to be a big deal?

It's an important conversation—one that can break the ice and set the relationship on a very positive course. Its outcome is not completely in your control. But there are things you can do to shape the message and the response.

MAKING THE CHOICE

As some people ponder having this kind of "heart-to-heart" with a lover or romantic interest, they begin to wonder if it's really necessary. Why risk rejection, they reason, when there may be another way? What about just avoiding sex during herpes outbreaks, and practicing safer sex in between?

Opening up about herpes can be intimidating, and certainly there are individuals who choose *not* to tell a sex partner about herpes or who find it impossible to tell until after they've had sex. There are countless combinations of people and circumstances, and no book such as this can presume to anticipate them all. In couples who pursue an ongoing relationship, however, it's clearly helpful if herpes isn't a secret locked away from your lover.

For one thing, the secrecy itself is likely to cause more anxiety than telling the truth. The closer you become, the more you'll want to be honest—yet the task at hand is likely to get harder over time. If and when you do finally disclose the truth, suddenly there are two issues on the table. One is herpes. But potentially more explosive is the issue of trust.

Withholding the truth poses other problems as well. It puts the entire burden of preventing the spread of herpes on one person. It may also lead to the adoption of unhealthy or irrational strategies to avert outbreaks or avoid sex, such as making up stories to explain away times when you cannot be intimate. These strategies themselves can be quite stressful and actually make having herpes more of a burden than it would otherwise be.

There also are ethical and legal implications. Everyone has the right to make an informed choice about his or her sexual partner, and the courts have ruled in some cases that failure to disclose a sexually transmitted infection like herpes may be grounds for a lawsuit. (These suits aren't common, but some individuals do choose to bring legal action.)

It's clear that keeping herpes secret from your lover can fuel emotional stress, but there are health-related issues at stake as well. Just as your partner may be at risk for herpes, he or she may place you at risk for a number of other STIs. *You* have something to gain from knowing your potential partner's sexual history, too. So it makes sense to talk about herpes in the context of overall sexual health. This approach equalizes people from the beginning. Remember also that about one-fifth of the adult population has herpes, though most don't know it. So a potential partner may have the same virus. (Herpes diagnostic tests for partners are discussed in Chapters 13 and 16.)

In reality, questions about risks to your health are relevant to both partners: Have you had another lover in the past? Have you used condoms? Have you ever had a sexually transmitted infection? Do you realize that you can have HIV or other STIs and not know it? These may be difficult issues to raise, but frank discussion about these things is becoming the norm in more relationships all the time.

Honesty and open communication not only pave the way for making smart choices about prevention, they also carry emotional benefits, not the least of which are mutual trust and respect. Sometimes the person who is newly diagnosed feels reluctant to tell anyone about herpes. But psychologists have found that telling a sexual partner is very important in making the adjustment to herpes and learning to cope with it. Herpes or no herpes, communication and sharing are two of the cornerstones for any successful relationship.

STARTING WITH YOURSELF

Once you've decided to tell a partner about herpes, it may prove helpful to think through the process and anticipate some of the potential issues.

First, it's important to consider whether you've come to terms with herpes yourself and accepted that it's not such an earth-shaking problem. There's little to gain from opening up to others about herpes if you're likely to characterize it in the most negative way or if you are still punishing yourself over it in some way.

Self-image is a relevant concern here. If herpes has radically altered the way you see yourself, it may be that the best first step is to consider why herpes is affecting you and then try to address the root of the problem. Perhaps a trusted friend or counselor could help you think through these issues.

Whether or not you find it necessary to assess your self-esteem in this way, it's a good idea to know the key facts about herpes and feel comfortable discussing them. Be prepared for a range of questions—some of them thought-provoking and some of them quite simple. You probably know a great deal by now, but you have to assume that your audience is starting from scratch.

PREPARING TO TELL: WHEN AND HOW

Each person will have a style and presentation that's unique, and no one should feel constrained to use a schedule or a script that just doesn't fit the situation. However you proceed, though, your attitude and your mood will have a great deal of influence on how the news is received. People tend to behave the way you expect them to behave, and a gloomy presentation may well increase the chance of a gloomy response. So the key is to be positive and be confident. Expect that your partner will be accepting and supportive. You are doing the right thing for both of you.

What's the best time? People who have shared their experiences through herpes support groups or the newsletters of the American Social Health Association's Herpes Resource Center tend to agree that it's usually best to allow a relationship to develop a bit before bringing up the subject. A conversation about sexual health is going to be easier if you have begun to feel comfortable with someone and safe about being honest.

If you do become interested in someone and begin to feel comfortable in the relationship, you can prepare yourself and look for logical opportunities to broach the subject. A television or newspaper report on sexual health infertility or AIDS, for instance—might naturally start a conversation about safer sex.

A passionate embrace, however, is definitely not the perfect opportunity it might seem to be. In the heat of a sexually charged moment, discussion of herpes or other STIs can be particularly awkward and frustrating. Your partner may be angry with you for spoiling the mood, and this may color the entire conversation. Likewise, it's probably best not to broach the subject en route to a romantic getaway.

Many people choose to plan carefully a time and place for the conversation. And the consensus is that talking to a partner about sexual history works best when both individuals feel good, are relaxed, and can devote their full attention to the conversation. The place should be private. It could be your own home or a quiet outdoor setting—anywhere that's relatively free of interruptions.

WHAT TO SAY

If you're worried about how to handle the situation, you may want to write down what amounts to a script and practice it. Knowing what to say and actually speaking the words in advance can make things easier when the time comes.

Clearly, people take countless approaches, but a number of common elements are often cited:

• Begin the conversation by pointing to the strengths of the relationship. For example: "I really feel I can trust you, and I'd like to tell you something very personal. Last year I found out I contracted genital herpes." Or: "I really enjoy being with you, and I'm starting to feel very safe with you. It seems possible we will want to be more intimate in the future, so I think it's time we talk about safer sex."

• In describing herpes, keep things in perspective. Stress that it's a common viral infection and that there's medication available to treat it. Many people like to make the comparison with cold sores, since these are acknowledged as a very minor concern. For example: "Have you ever had a cold sore or a fever blister? The reason I ask is that cold sores are caused by a type of virus—herpes simplex virus. I have this virus, only for me instead of causing a sore on the lips, it can cause one below the waist."

• Mention that most people have either HSV-1 or HSV-2, and about one in five adults has genital herpes. It's usually so mild, however, that many people don't know they have it. Even people who have received a "clean bill of health" from a doctor or STI clinic may have undiagnosed genital herpes, since the use of accurate tests for herpes is not routine.

• In the interest of full disclosure, explain that herpes can be spread during sexual contact when sores or other symptoms are present. There may also be a risk of transmission at other times, but a person can take precautions to lower this risk.

Whatever the script, it's crucial to avoid being over-dramatic. Your delivery affects your message. Try to be calm and confident, straightforward and sincere. Frame the conversation the way you've decided to, and avoid language that's inherently negative. Lastly, don't lose sight of the fact that you want a dialogue, so it's best not to go on at great length. You want to discuss the issue, not lecture or confess.

Some may simply need time to process what you've said. Other times the first response is an attempt to sort out the information, and some people will want to read something on herpes, such as a brochure or book. Remember: You may have known very little about herpes before you were diagnosed. In any case, you have everything to gain from helping to provide information. You can also give a partner the telephone number of the National Herpes Hotline.

Having a partner take matters under advisement or go elsewhere for information isn't easy, but it's reasonable to expect that someone who is new to the idea of herpes may need time to absorb the facts and check their own feelings. And the outcome can be very satisfying, as in the case of Lauren. "I contracted herpes five years ago from a partner who failed to tell me that he had it," she says. "I have slowly come to terms with my anger towards him and myself. Since that time, I have been sexually active with two different men. Each time, I *chose* to talk about herpes before getting sexually involved. In each case, my boyfriend decided that herpes should not get in the way of having a sexual relationship. Both needed time or needed to read something before making a decision, and one consulted his doctor. My point is simply that it may take some patience, but you can have this conversation and have it turn out well."

Also, remain open to the possibility that the person you're talking to may have herpes themselves. In describing herpes, you may have cited the fact that herpes goes unrecognized most of the time. The person you're telling may be one of those who has this type of unrecognized infection. In approaching the subject, make sure the person understands you are not implying he or she has herpes already or accusing them of withholding information from you. On the other hand, if the relationship progresses, getting a type-specific blood test for herpes can establish whether you and your potential partner already have the same type of HSV. If so, you have basically eliminated transmission as a concern. We'll discuss these tests and their use further in Chapter 13 and Chapter 16.

Clearly, if there are countless approaches, there are an equal number of subtleties in the responses you might get. Some people may overreact, some won't bat an eye. Given the number of people who have herpes, many will have had this discussion before. Whatever the reaction, try to be flexible yourself. Remember that it took you time to adjust as well, and that the first response is not always the one that counts.

At the same time, some experts say, don't be overly concerned about protecting the feelings of your partner. Yes, you want him or her to have the time needed to process this information. But after all, you have needs yourself. And you probably don't need a relationship in which you have to do all the emotional work. Has your partner given you a feeling of emotional support? It's important to assess the other person's behavior when presented with the challenge of a safer sex discussion. People who are judgmental, those who have a very narrow life experience, or those who are obsessive about germs may not be the best candidates for your love.

The majority of people will react well. After all, you trust them enough to share a confidence with them that you probably wouldn't share with just anybody. Most people respect that. And in talking about safer sex, you've shown maturity in facing up to a health issue of mutual importance for any two people So, when you talk to someone about herpes and safer sex, pat yourself on the back. You have confronted a difficult issue in your life with courage and consideration.

MANAGING HERPES

13

HERPES AND YOUR SEX LIFE

⟋◎⟍

"I've been in a relationship with Jeff for several months," says Denise. "At first I didn't know how to tell him I had herpes, but through an unplanned conversation about past lovers and STIs he learned about it. He has been very understanding and supportive. Jeff has not wanted to be tested so far, so we're still taking precautions. I'm on daily suppressive therapy, and I'm kind of insisting he use condoms so that he's protected—although I don't know how much longer he is going to want to do that."

People worry about the effect herpes is going to have on their sex life. It's one of the concerns that can make herpes seem so difficult initially, and it's central to the anxiety over telling a partner. Starting or maintaining an intimate relationship isn't the easiest thing in the world, anyway. And putting herpes into the mix may add an unwanted layer of complexity.

In assessing its likely impact on one's sex life, it's useful to remember that herpes affects everyone differently at an emotional level. For some, it's a minor matter. For others, it can cause a number of concerns, including problems of self-esteem or feelings of isolation. Sexually, it can affect one's sense of spontaneity or freedom. Some may feel more hesitant to approach new partners or may experience a decrease in sexual pleasure around the time of diagnosis—feelings that often center on the fear of spreading herpes to a partner. These concerns may be heightened if the person is experiencing frequent outbreaks.

As with other aspects of genital herpes, however, such concerns tend to be especially pressing in the first few months after being diagnosed. Later, they tend to fade. In fact, one study found that there were no long-term changes in the sex lives of persons diagnosed with herpes, compared with the period before diagnosis.

Talking about the lessening impact of herpes over the long-term is not to trivialize it or deny that it may bring some changes to your sex life. The most important of these is probably the issue of risk reduction—of protecting sexual partners.

The desire to protect a sexual partner and prevent the spread of herpes is often very strong. In a number of different studies, a very high percentage of people with herpes listed fear of infecting a partner as one of their primary concerns. In this chapter we'll take a detailed look at the factors that increase or lower the risk of transmitting herpes and at the steps you can take to reduce this risk in your relationships. We'll also review considerations that may influence these choices, such as the possibility that your sexual partner wants to be tested for herpes. Testing, after all, can color this entire discussion. If you and a partner have the same type of HSV, the risk of transmission becomes moot and the precautions listed here may be irrelevant in this particular relationship.

THE BASICS

First we'll focus on herpes by itself. Forget about whether you're gay or straight, coupled or single; forget about the other STIs. In the absence of all other factors, what you can do to prevent the spread of herpes boils down to three steps:

1. Avoid direct skin-to-skin contact with herpes lesions during obvious flare-ups.
2. Use risk reduction. Both daily valacyclovir and condoms can be used between outbreaks as a guard against the asymptomatic shedding discussed in earlier chapters. For oral sex protection, use a dental dam, a condom cut in half, or a sheet of plastic wrap. (See pages 147-150.)
3. Discuss HSV with your partner. Research shows that transmission is more likely when disclosure of herpes has been avoided. Plus, when it comes to making decisions about condoms or other risk reduction strategies, an open conversation is the healthiest option.

The first two of these steps center on times when HSV has reactivated and caused the process of viral shedding. As we have discussed, shedding rates are highly variable. Because they are also largely unpredictable, the precautions needed to protect a partner deserve a detailed discussion.

During Outbreaks

The risk of spreading herpes is highest whenever symptoms, ranging from subtle to painful, are present. The tingling or itch of prodrome, for example, is a signal that virus has probably found its way to the skin and that there is risk of spreading HSV to a sexual partner. An itchy red patch of skin near the genitals also should be considered a likely site of viral shedding, as should a classic herpes lesion. Herpes can be spread when any such signs and symptoms are present.

Sometimes a person may experience the symptoms of prodrome and then have no visible signs of infection at all. This is sometimes called a "false prodrome," but it can just as easily be regarded as a minor outbreak. You should still consider that the risk of transmission is high when the itching or tingling sensations occur, because the virus may be present on your skin at this time.

When signs and symptoms are present, any direct genital-to-genital contact or sexual act that involves penetration, such as vaginal or anal sex, creates a high risk of transmission. Also included as risky would be oral-to-genital contact (mouth on vaginal area or mouth on penis).

When can you consider an outbreak over? The basic rule is to avoid direct contact with the affected area from the first hint of prodrome until any skin lesions are fully healed and the skin surface looks normal again. In some cases, this is a matter of days. With recurrences, the process takes 4 to 6 days on average; with a first episode, it may be quite a bit longer. Studies have shown that asymptomatic shedding is most probable in the days immediately before or after an outbreak, so after herpes lesions heal—even after a scab falls off—it's safest to leave the tender new skin alone for a few days.

What about simply using condoms during outbreaks? Unfortunately, condoms do not offer complete protection during these periods. There are a variety of possible reasons for this. Incorrect or inconsistent use is certainly a major factor. (A list of condom do's and don'ts is included later in this chapter.) In addition, in terms of simple geography, some herpes lesions will be covered or protected by a condom, but some will not. A herpes lesion on the upper thigh, for example, will not be covered. Alternately, if a woman were having a lesion in the folds of the vulva or in the perianal area, it's unclear whether the use of a condom by a male partner would provide complete coverage and protection.

All of this would be much simpler, too, if an outbreak were always a matter of a lesion you could clearly see. In reality, however, during recurrences HSV may travel to several skin sites at once. There may be an obvious lesion in one place—say, on the penis— and asymptomatic shedding in another.

In summary, condoms might help reduce the risk of transmission during outbreaks, depending on the circumstances. But they are not a guarantee of protection—especially when symptoms are present.

While the risk of spreading herpes is high when lesions are present, some couples find creative ways to give one another pleasure without taking large risks. First, as long as there are no lesions on the mouth, kissing poses no risk. Sensual massage, mutual masturbation, fantasy—all these are sexual practices that some people recount using as forms of risk reduction, and many say they are quite pleasurable.

Many people wonder about risks involved in use of the hands for sexual pleasuring. No form of skin-to-skin contact with a herpes lesion is absolutely risk free. For example, HSV could be transferred from a site of viral shedding to an uninfected partner during love-making by way of the hand. In a ranking of risks, use of the hands is probably safer than genital-to-genital contact or oral sex, because the thick skin of the hands is less vulnerable to HSV. When lesions are present, however, concern about transmission via the hands is warranted.

Refraining from intercourse isn't easy sometimes, and in one recent study, about one-fifth of couples in monogamous relationships reported that they sometimes chose to have intercourse when lesions were present. It's clear, however, that a greater number of exposures to herpes lesions increases the risk of transmission. Therefore, couples who refrain from sexual intercourse during outbreaks are taking an important step to avoid spreading herpes from one to the other.

Between Outbreaks

Even if you have outbreaks more often than the average person, the vast majority of your days will be symptom-free. The problem is the issue of asymptomatic viral shedding.

As we noted in Chapters 5 and 6, asymptomatic shedding occurs in all persons who have genital HSV-2, at rates that vary from person to person. As measured by viral culture tests, the *average* person sheds on something like 4% of days (something on the order of 15 to 20 days per year), and the rate is significantly higher with the more sensitive PCR test. The real problem is, you don't know which days these will be.

What can you do about it? Let's look in more detail at the major risk reduction strategies:

SUPPRESSIVE ANTIVIRAL MEDICATION: You have already read in Chapter 9 about the transmission study conducted with a daily regimen of suppressive valacyclovir. This research proved the concept that antiviral activity really does translate to a reduced risk of spreading herpes. Specifically, individuals with recurrent genital HSV-2 could take 500 mg of valacyclovir once a day and cut the risk of transmission in half. Though not perfect, suppressive therapy with valacyclovir is an important prevention option that patients did not have until just recently. The FDA has labeled the drug for use in preventing heterosexual transmission in persons with healthy immune systems. The CDC's 2006 treatment guidelines state that it is likely to be effective also for other immune-competent individuals, including men who have sex with men. It is not known whether other dosages of valacyclovir or acyclovir might work as well or better. However, for persons who are able to take a medication twice a day, acyclovir twice daily or valacyclovir twice daily results in a slightly better control of genital herpes recurrences, and perhaps of viral shedding as well.

CONDOMS: For straight or gay couples practicing vaginal or anal intercourse, use of male condoms between herpes outbreaks is another solid option. You recall that condoms were *not* recommended as protection *during* outbreaks, but they're considered a better bet for asymptomatic shedding. Why? Research to date suggests that the biggest risk of asymptomatic transmission occurs when there is contact between surfaces such as the penis or the soft mucosal tissue of the vagina, cervix, or anus. And these, of course, are among the areas that *tend to be* covered or protected by condoms.

The best overall data we have about condoms comes from a recent vaccine study, which followed several hundred couples over a period of time and documented each instance where herpes was spread from one partner to the other. In this study, condom use was quite low in spite of the fact that all participants were counseled to use them consistently. But various analyses of the data on condom use show that those who used condoms for the largest percentage of sexual acts had a significantly reduced risk of transmission. Researchers say the bottom line is approximately a 50% reduction in risk for both men and women—essentially equivalent to the protection given by antiviral therapy. (See page 147 for information about condom types and safe use.)

So, what about condoms and suppressive valacyclovir together? Sadly, it's difficult to draw any conclusions about this question. Rates of condom use in the valacyclovir transmission study were quite low, despite the counseling message that condoms should be used. Condom use is also very low in other recent studies on transmission risk. Therefore, researchers lack the data to tease apart the relative effectiveness of condoms versus antiviral therapy. If you are intent on doing everything you can to lower the risk of transmission, using both approaches makes a lot of sense.

TALKING IT OVER: It might seem like a stretch to say that telling a partner about herpes is a form of risk reduction, but research data make it clear that this kind of disclosure is associated with a reduced risk of transmission. A 2006 study of 199 individuals attending a Seattle STI clinic carefully examined the various risk factors that might contribute to acquiring herpes. Researchers looked closely at certain variables in the relationships between the study subjects and the transmitting partner. Among those whose partners had not disclosed the fact they had genital herpes, the median time to transmission was 60 days. In those who did disclose, it was 270 days.

Also relevant here is the fact that open communication is optimal for negotiating issues like whether and how often to use condoms, or whether it's a good idea for a new partner to get tested for HSV-2 to see if they might already have the virus anyway.

RISK REDUCTION FOR GAYS AND LESBIANS

The data that have been gathered about the transmission of herpes stem primarily from research on heterosexual couples, but gays and lesbians often raise questions about the particular risks they may face. In addition, many people—both straight and gay—are eager to learn whether anything is known about the relative risks of various sexual acts.

Unfortunately, medical science has little to say about the probability of transmission through oral sex versus anal sex versus other types of sexual pleasuring. But there are some insights about herpes that may be particularly pertinent for gays and for lesbians.

Given the enormous impact of AIDS, people in the gay community are better informed about HIV prevention than most other segments of the U.S. population. The importance of herpes and other STIs as risk factors for acquiring HIV, however, has not always been well publicized. Specifically, research has shown that genital herpes—and, in fact, a number of other STIs—create tiny breaks in the skin and in mucosal tissue that give HIV a portal of entry. In addition, herpes lesions attract larger than average numbers of T cells—precisely the kind of lymphocyte that HIV likes to attack. Given these two factors, the person who is experiencing a herpes outbreak or an episode of asymptomatic shedding has an especially high risk of getting infected with HIV if he or she is exposed to HIV. The "if" here is important, because it is not true that herpes puts one on some inevitable path to HIV, but the added risk of HIV is worth considering. For similar reasons, those who are HIV-positive and also have genital herpes are likely more efficient transmitters of both HIV and HSV.

All of the above argues for the same kinds of precautions outlined previously, such as abstaining from sex during outbreaks and condom use at other times. Condoms have been studied more thoroughly for their efficacy in vaginal sex, but for over a decade the CDC has been recommending their use for anal and oral sex as well. For both vaginal and anal sex, water-based lubricants will likely offer an extra measure of protection, decreasing the likelihood of condom breakage and of trauma to the rectum that can result from anal inter-course.

By comparison with gay men, lesbians have been regarded as unlikely to acquire STIs such as herpes and HIV. But while the rates of some STIs are indeed lower in lesbians, a study at the University of Washington showed that some 13% of lesbian women tested posi-tive for HSV-2. How do they acquire it? First, researchers point out that as many as 90% of women who identify themselves as lesbian have had sex with men at some point in their lives. Second, given the importance of oral sex in lesbian couples, it's likely that HSV is some-times spread through oral-genital contact, and likely as well that there is a fairly high percentage of HSV-1 in lesbian women that represents latent genital infection. Third, women who have sex with women may be able to transmit STIs such as genital HPV—and possibly herpes—through sex toys and through use of the hands for pleasur-ing.

In terms of prevention, researchers stress that women who have sex with women should be aware that oral sex does pose a risk of transmission. In this regard, as a barrier during oral sex, some women use a dental dam or household plastic wrap as a protective barrier. Some use nonpowdered latex gloves, which can be cut to a suitable flat shape for covering the vulva. As far as sex toys, it's important to understand that viruses or bacteria deposited on the toy by one person can infect the other during penetration or rubbing. The best advice, therefore, is to clean them with soap and water before sharing.

SELF-IMAGE AND SEXUAL GROWTH

A great deal has been written on the mechanics of "safer sex." A lot of it, unfortunately, doesn't get to the heart of the matter for many people who have recently been diagnosed and are feeling very threatened by the potential changes in their sexual habits.

In an ASHA survey, for example, many respondents noted ways in which herpes affected their sense of sexual spontaneity or freedom. Some felt more hesitant to approach new partners, while a few withdrew from sexual activity for months or even years. Two out of three said they experienced a decrease in sexual pleasure around the time of diagnosis. And almost as many reported that herpes lessened sexual drive during outbreaks. Similar results were found in a number of studies over the past two decades.

As with other aspects of genital herpes, however, for many individuals the impact on sexuality lessens markedly over time. One researcher noted that after a period of six months, persons diagnosed with herpes were enjoying sex just as much as they did before and functioned just as they had before. In the short-term, however, one may experience a sense of loss in having to feel more constrained in one's sex life. Frequently, a period of adjustment may be needed.

At the same time, it can be very damaging to conclude that you're no longer a sexual person or no longer allowed to express sexual desire. STIs such as herpes sometimes have the seeming power to overwhelm us and become what psychologists call "master status traits." Thus, our sexual self-image can undergo a change because of a medical condition.

If you're feeling this way, it may be important to keep sight of the fact that millions of people with herpes do have satisfying sexual relationships. When questioned about the long-term impact of herpes, counselors and sex therapists point out that a condition like genital herpes can actually have a very positive effect on relationships. Talking through an issue like herpes can create a deeper level of trust and intimacy, and some couples say that herpes influences them to explore and grow sexually.

Herpes can press couples to communicate about what is sexually pleasing. And that's no small accomplishment, because people in all sorts of relationships often have trouble talking about sex. Needs and desires remain unspoken out of embarrassment. But being forced to speak about them can have unforeseen benefits and result in more mature and more creative sex.

An easy way to begin communicating about sex is to tell your partner you want to talk about it. Talking about "talking about" sex can lead a couple to share their fears and feelings. They may then be comfortable enough to begin an ongoing process of sexual communication.

Says one therapist: "I've had clients who have had to deal with severe herpes outbreaks over time. But it's not really an issue. A satisfying sexuality really has more to do with being comfortable with sexuality in general, being able to talk about it with your partner, and being willing to try new things with your partner. Healthy sexuality has more to do with the couple's *attitude* about sex than it has to do with an issue such as herpes."

If all the talk about condoms puts you off, or if you've been diagnosed recently and are just not ready to become sexually active, remember two things: First, it may take a while before you feel yourself again, but you're still a whole and healthy individual who can have satisfying sexual relationships. Second, you may discover new aspects of your sexuality because of herpes.

Some choose to date other people with herpes, at least as a way of getting started on dating again. This can ease the problem of having to disclose herpes to a partner and may have other advantages as well. With the popularity of online dating services, there are a number of dating sites that actually specialize in herpes and make it easy to con-

nect to a community of people who have the shared experience of a
herpes diagnosis. That said, we stress that this isn't for everyone, and
no one should feel that getting herpes has redefined their social net-
work or identity.

THINKING THROUGH THE ISSUES:
TESTING, RISK, AND CHOICES

Faced with all this information, many people understand-
ably have a hard time knowing what to do about herpes and sex.
Unfortunately, this book can't provide any easy answers or foolproof
formulas. Every person has a unique situation and unique set of values, and decisions about sex hinge on both.

In addition, it's worth mentioning again that, while people with
herpes may be highly concerned about their partners, they should
not be oblivious to the need to protect themselves from other, poten
tially more serious sexually transmitted infections. As we've said,
there are 19 million new sexually transmitted infections each year,
and some experts say that 50% of adults—whatever their race, sex,
or social class—will have an STI at some point. Many of these infections can remain hidden, so that those who carry them don't know
about it. The point is that while protecting a partner is often the
focal point for safer sex practices, the person with herpes should not
overlook his or her own risk. In many circumstances, personal risk
will or should influence one's decision, for example, on condom use.

TESTING: In terms of protecting a partner against herpes, the
first issue is: Does your partner possibly have herpes already? As
we mentioned earlier, this may not be an easy matter to bring up,
and you would want to avoid any implication that your partner

is withholding something from you. However, if your partner has learned the basics about herpes, understands how widespread it is, and understands that up to 85% of those who have antibodies don't recognize symptoms, then it may make sense to talk about testing. If the two of you agree that it's important to find out, your partner (and possibly you) can get one of the new "type-specific" blood tests for HSV. Finding an accurate test and learning more about how to interpret the test are two topics covered in detail in Chapter 16.

In cases where two partners both have some form of HSV, various questions can arise. If the partners both have genital HSV-2, for example, is there any need for precautions? For the most part, no—issues of prevention are a largely a moot point. In this scenario, experts would still recommend avoiding sex when symptoms are present, because it's possible—though unlikely—to be reinfected with a different strain of HSV-2. But, even here, the chance of this resulting in a greater number of outbreaks is very small.

What if one person has a history of type 1 herpes (let's say it's cold sores) and the other a history of genital HSV-2? Will each of them become infected with both types? And will they have more frequent recurrences as a result?

The research on this question has produced contradictory findings. Some studies suggest that the person with pre-existing HSV-1 infection has a lower risk of acquiring HSV-2. Other studies suggest no such protection. But the consensus among researchers is that people with HSV-1 who later acquire HSV-2 will, *at a minimum*, have milder clinical signs and symptoms than those who acquire HSV-2 without prior HSV-1.

If we turn the tables and ask about HSV-2, the answer is more definitive. It's clear that the person with pre-existing HSV-2 *does* have some protection against HSV-1. So the body's natural defenses will certainly be relevant in this scenario. The bottom line is that type-specific testing will offer some important information.

In addition, one might weigh the "sites of preference" data. That is, if one becomes infected with genital HSV-1, it's known that recurrences are less frequent than they are with genital HSV-2. And while HSV-1 recurs around the face with some regularity, recurrences of oral HSV-2 are quite uncommon.

ASSESSING RISK REDUCTION: If testing is not an option, or if you discover that your partner does not have herpes, there are several aspects of risk reduction to consider. First, some people are curious to understand the risk statistically, but this may vary over the period of the relationship. In addition, it's hard to set the basis for acceptable risk. A risk of 1 in 10 may be acceptable to one person, while a risk of 1 in 100 may be unacceptable to another. In general, younger individuals are at higher risk, and so are persons in casual, short-term relationships. One of the most significant factors, however, is gender. The best data suggest that women are two to three times as likely as men to become infected with herpes if exposed to the virus. A similar increase in risk to women is noted with several other STIs as well. At least in part, this is probably due to the physical differences between the sexes—mainly the presence of more mucosal tissue in women.

Recent research has turned up new insights into other risk factors as well. It appears that risk of transmission is highest when the person with herpes has both HSV-1 and HSV-2. Risk is also increased *early* in the course of any sexual relationship. The most obvious explanation for this is the fact that couples tend to have sex more often early in the relationship, and the number of exposures correlates with increased risk. Some scientists also theorize that transmission rates are higher early on because people vary in how easily they get the infection. In this hypothesis, the first year may sort out the "susceptibles" from those who are not.

These epidemiological facts might be useful, but at the end of the day everyone is faced with the same basic challenge. If your partner does not have antibodies to HSV—or specifically to the type you have—there is some risk of transmission from asymptomatic shedding. The best prescription for lowering risk is to have an honest discussion about the options. Taking suppressive valacyclovir and using condoms between outbreaks would be the most thorough approach, but this won't fit every couple's situation.

In some relationships, risk reduction won't be a major issue. You may have a partner who knows there is a chance of becoming infected and simply is not worried about it. Alternately, you may find your partner has the same type of HSV already. Some couples in long-term relationships find that they are less concerned about the possibility of transmission as time goes on.

In the end, genital herpes doesn't have to stand in the way of having a healthy and satisfying sex life. Taking precautions to protect your partner—and to protect yourself from other STIs—is something that more and more people are learning to negotiate. There are as many different approaches as there are people.

USING CONDOMS

When it comes to STI protection, any condom is better than none, but condoms made of latex or plastic (polyurethane and other synthetic materials) are better than those made of animal membrane. "Lambskin" or animal-membrane condoms have pores large enough to admit some viruses—at least in laboratory experiments—and are not recommended for STI protection. But even the smallest viruses cannot permeate latex or plastic.

Condoms sold for contraception and disease protection in this country are classified as medical devices. They are regulated by the U.S. Food and Drug Administration and carefully tested and inspected during the manufacturing process. Every latex condom sold in the U.S. is tested electronically for holes before packaging. Condom failure usually results from inconsistent or incorrect use rather than condom breakage.

Latex is recommended by public health authorities as the preferred type of condom for STI protection. In randomized, controlled studies, plastic condoms have been shown to be three to five times more likely to break than latex condoms. Research suggests men are generally more satisfied with the latex condom as well, though some individuals may prefer non-latex condoms or need to use them because of latex allergies.

THE BASICS — If you are starting to use condoms for the first time, it's important to review the package insert or other written instructions about how to use them correctly. The basics are as follows: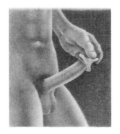

• Check to see that the condom package is not torn or damaged. Also check the expiration date on the package. *(Latex condoms have a shelf life of 3 to 5 years.)* Never use a condom that is brittle, dry, or has changed color.

• Condoms should be stored in a cool, dry place out of direct sunlight—no wallets or glove compartments.

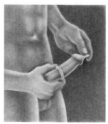

• Put the condom on before any genital contact occurs. If the condom has a reservoir tip, squeeze the tip closed and unroll the condom onto the erect penis. Air bubbles may lead to breakage.

• If the condom does not have a reservoir tip, hold the end of the condom between the thumb and the forefinger and unroll the condom onto the erect penis. This should leave extra room at the tip of the condom *(to hold semen after ejaculation).*

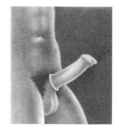

• Unroll the condom to cover the entire erect penis. The unrolled ring should be on the outside. If the condom is on inside out, do not flip it over. It might have pre-ejaculation fluid on it. Use another condom.

• *If the condom is latex*, only water-based lubricants should be used *(K-Y® Brand Jelly, Replens®, or Astroglide®, for example)*. Oil-based lubricants can damage latex, so do not usc Vaseline® petroleum jelly, baby oil, vegetable oil, or most hand and skin lotions.

• *If the condom is plastic,* the oil-based lubricants mentioned above will not degrade the material.

• Following ejaculation, while the penis is still erect, hold the base of the condom and withdraw, taking care not to let the condom slip off. A condom should never be used twice.

Condoms can be used for various sexual activities. They are tested under conditions that simulate vaginal intercourse, but many experts consider them effective for oral sex and anal sex as well. Condoms can be used with or without lubricant. Many brands are coated with lubricant at the factory, though unlubricated brands are also available. Because many people object to the smell and taste of latex, some manufacturers also market flavored condoms specifically for use in oral sex.

THE FEMALE CONDOM — In fact, because of the emphasis on safer sex beginning in the late 1980s, condom manufacturers developed diverse product lines. In addition to the plastic condom recently developed for men, there are a number of condoms designed to be used by women. One type of female condom (branded as FC or FC2 Female Condom®) is a plastic 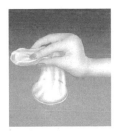 pouch with a flexible loop on either end. The smaller of the two loops is inserted in the vagina, covering the cervix, and the larger loop lies outside, covering the vulva. It was hoped this model might actually offer greater protection against STIs than the standard male condom because it covers more area. However, so far we have no conclusive evidence that it is more protective. In any case, it gives women an option they can initiate. Some women whose partners cannot or will not use latex condoms are able to use the female condom.

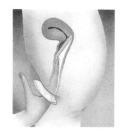

SPERMICIDES? NO. — People concerned about safer sex often ask questions about spermicide as well. The active ingredient in foams, jellies, and suppositories used by some women to prevent pregnancy also kills or

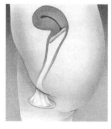

disables certain viruses and bacteria. Currently, however, the Centers for Disease Control and Prevention does not recommend use of spermicides for prevention of HIV or other STIs because of studies that show regular spermicide use may cause tissue damage that actually increases risk.

OTHER STI PROTECTION

DENTAL DAM — A dental dam is a small, thin, square piece of latex that is used for oral-vaginal or oral-anal sex. (Also used in dental procedures.) Dental dams help to reduce the transmission of herpes and other STIs during oral sex by acting as a barrier to vaginal and anal secretions that contain bacteria and viruses. Be sure to use one side only. Sold in pharmacies, sex stores and online, they come in a variety of sizes and flavors. (Note: A condom cut in half lengthwise or a square of plastic wrap can also provide protection for oral sex.)

14

HERPES AND PREGNANCY

"After having several outbreaks a year, I got pregnant with my first child," writes Marilu. *"And deep down I was really worried. Childbirth was the one thing about herpes that always seemed scary to me. Even so, despite tremendous stress during pregnancy (changing jobs and moving), I had only one outbreak. I delivered vaginally after a long and painful labor. My baby and I were treated with kind and loving care, and after a two-day stay, we went home."*

Even people who have learned to manage genital herpes with ease often have concerns about pregnancy and their ability to give birth to a healthy child. On one hand, these worries are reasonable, because HSV infection in a newborn can be a devastating illness. On the other hand, this kind of herpes infection is quite rare. Out of approximately 4 million live births every year in the United States, the number of babies contracting neonatal herpes is estimated at between 400 and 2800. In many cases, these babies are born to women who contract herpes late in pregnancy, rather than to women who have long-standing infections. What's more, women who have genital herpes and recognize it can take precautions to lower the already small risk that their infants might become infected.

HOW HSV CAN SPREAD TO NEWBORNS

Transmission of genital HSV to newborns follows the same basic principles that govern transmission between adults and is most likely to occur during labor and delivery. If HSV reactivates in a pregnant woman around the time of labor, it's likely that she will be shedding virus somewhere in the birth canal. Fully developed herpes lesions pose the greatest threat to the infant; therefore, if a woman has signs and symptoms of active herpes infection at labor, precautions are usually taken to protect the baby from infection. Asymptomatic shedding may also pose a risk, especially if it occurs during a first episode.

While the vast majority of transmission from mother to infant takes place at birth, there are two other possibilities. First, researchers believe that in very rare cases a fetus may become infected during pregnancy, especially if the mother has a primary episode during pregnancy. The theory is that a large amount of HSV can be present in the mother's body, including her blood, and some of it may cross the placenta or find its way into the amniotic fluid. Second, infants can become infected *after* birth if an adult with active herpes lesions transmits HSV through direct contact. The classic example of this is the relative who has an active cold sore and kisses a baby.

ASSESSING THE RISK

Research on neonatal herpes conducted during the 1980s and 1990s has shed a great deal of light on the question of which deliveries carry the highest risk. It turns out that more than half of the babies infected with herpes at delivery are born to mothers who acquired genital herpes in the last trimester of pregnancy. Some of these women actually had herpes lesions but did not realize it and were not adequately examined before giving birth. Others may have been shedding virus asymptomatically as a result of a first episode. If this seems hard to believe, remember that most people with genital herpes don't know they have it.

What about women who have had herpes for a long time? Here, too, there is a need for careful medical management. In rare cases, babies can become infected when exposed to asymptomatic viral shedding in the birth canal of mothers who have recurrent genital herpes. In this situation, the risk of transmission to the newborn is quite small—probably less than .01%. When a woman with recurrent herpes has an outbreak at the time of delivery, the risk is much less than with a first episode, but it's still high enough that medical experts recommend delivery by cesarean section (C-section).

Why is there such a dramatic difference in the risks posed by these two categories of herpes infection? A herpes infection in a pregnant woman who has never before been infected with HSV-1 or HSV-2 raises the level of risk for four reasons:

1. Neither mother nor infant will have antibodies to HSV.
2. More virus is present in a first episode than in a recurrent outbreak.
3. The cervix is more often involved in a first episode, which means the baby has a greater chance of coming into contact with virus in the birth canal.
4. The virus remains active for a longer period in a first episode.

The relative contribution of each of these factors is not known, but all are thought to play a role in compounding the risk of neonatal infection.

Babies born to women with a history of genital herpes, on the other hand, have a major advantage over those born to women who first become infected with HSV during pregnancy. Nature offers significant protection to these infants by giving them HSV antibodies while they're still in the womb. These antibodies come directly from the mother and cross the placenta in the blood supply to the fetus. There they can protect the baby from acquiring infection during birth, even if there is virus in the birth canal. Over the first six months of life, as the baby develops its own immune system, these antibodies are gradually lost. Recurrent infection is associated with fewer lesions and is less likely to involve the cervix, and the period of viral shedding is also likely to be shorter than during a first infection.

PREVENTION: WOMEN WITH RECURRENT HERPES

If you are pregnant and have a history of recurrent genital herpes (or recurrent genital symptoms you think may be herpes), the first step is to discuss your medical history with your doctor or midwife. With this information on the table, you and your healthcare provider can make plans for a number of contingencies that may arise if you have an outbreak near the time of labor and delivery. An open discussion of this issue can also help you emotionally by quelling any anxieties you may feel about herpes and an ill-timed recurrence.

The standard of care is to proceed with a normal vaginal delivery if a woman has no signs or symptoms of an outbreak. If, on the other hand, a woman with recurrent genital herpes has visible lesions or other symptoms of active infection at the time of labor, the baby is delivered by C-section. In this way, the baby is spared the risk of traveling through a birth canal where HSV might be present.

If you normally get outbreaks from time to time, you can expect to have some during your pregnancy, particularly in the third trimester. Herpes outbreaks sometimes increase in frequency as pregnancy progresses. There is also a higher than average risk of asymptomatic shedding late in pregnancy. Unfortunately, it is not possible to predict whether the shedding will occur at the time of labor.

As a precaution against HSV reactivation, a visual pelvic examination is recommended early in labor to look for herpes lesions. Experts point out that in many cases the obstetrician might not be present until late in labor, when the woman's cervix is almost fully dilated. Even then, the standard in many institutions is a quick manual examination. This may prove a case of "too little, too late," because a thorough visual exam with adequate light may be needed to detect herpes lesions. Thus, the need for a visual exam is one of the key issues to bring up with your obstetrician or midwife.

Another point for discussion with your obstetric healthcare provider is C-section delivery. Some women with genital herpes become so concerned about a safe delivery that they urge their doctor or midwife to opt for C section, and some doctors are inclined to recommend it for similar reasons. Even when herpes lesions are not present, professional concern over malpractice suits also contributes to the high rate of C-sections for women with genital herpes. However, leading experts agree that a woman with a history of genital herpes should deliver her baby vaginally unless symptoms (including prodromal symptoms) or herpes sores are present. C-section, they believe, is not needed unless some other complication of pregnancy is also present. The issue is that a C-section itself carries a substantial risk and a high cost. It is major surgery that entails the health risks of anesthesia, costs several thousand dollars more than a vaginal delivery, involves a longer and more complicated period of recovery, and frequently results in cesarean deliveries for subsequent births.

In planning for the birth of your baby, it's also important to know the policies of your chosen hospital or birthing center. Some hospitals have very strict procedures for isolating patients whose pregnancy is complicated by infectious disease. Such isolation policies are no longer recommended by herpes experts, but you would be well advised to ask in advance. If the hospital you've chosen has rules that conflict with your plans (plans to "room in," for example), you might want to consider having your baby at a different institution.

Many women wonder about the advisability of taking an antiviral drug during pregnancy. In general, it is recommended that women do not take medicines during pregnancy, especially during the first trimester, unless the benefits and risks are carefully considered. While no drug against herpes is specifically approved for use in pregnancy by the FDA, severe outbreaks are often treated with acyclovir, much as they would be treated at other times. In addition, some experts recommend the use of antiviral drugs in the last month of pregnancy to prevent outbreaks and asymptomatic shedding near the time of labor. Studies suggest that acyclovir taken daily after 36 weeks of gestation will reduce the likelihood of genital herpes recurrences and, therefore, decrease the need for C-sections. The prodrug valacyclovir is also used. Advocates of suppressive therapy in the last month of pregnancy believe it is best to increase the usual dosages used for suppression, to compensate for a change in the way antiviral drugs are metabolized by the pregnant woman. Guidelines for treatment during pregnancy are still being debated in the medical community, with some clinicians remaining concerned about the safety of fetal exposure to antiviral drugs.

Besides those cases in which acyclovir has been deliberately prescribed during pregnancy, some women have used it inadvertently before realizing they were expecting. A voluntary registry that tracked both kinds of exposure—more than 1,000 cases—saw no indication that the drug is harmful to mother or child. While there is not enough evidence to pronounce the drug categorically safe in pregnancy, acyclovir is one of the few that has been subject to systematic study in pregnant women.

A related concern that might arise is treatment of women who *acquire* herpes late in pregnancy, the scenario that creates a high risk of neonatal infection. As we explained earlier in this Chapter, the risk is elevated here due to the large amount of virus present and the lack of antibody in the woman during the initial infection. (Remember: The body's immune response to herpes takes several months to become established, during which time neither mother nor baby has the protection of HSV antibodies.) Because of the large quantities of virus involved in a first episode—and the likelihood of significant viral shedding in the birth canal—it is critical that women experiencing first episodes of genital herpes during the third trimester receive prompt antiviral treatment. The goal of treatment in such cases is to reduce the risk of viral shedding. Most experts also recommend C-section delivery *prior to rupture of membranes* for women who acquire HSV in late pregnancy in order to limit the baby's potential exposure. In addition, after delivery, some expert clinicians would start the baby on antiviral therapy until they have test results that confirm the baby is not infected.

One other issue worth mentioning centers on labor itself: The use of fetal scalp monitors. In the largest study to date on herpes and pregnancy, researchers at the University of Washington found that use of this type of monitor appeared to increase the risk of infection. The reason, probably, is that these instruments cause a tiny puncture in the scalp of the fetus, offering a possible opening for virus to enter.

The study results weren't statistically conclusive, but experts believe that for women with a history of genital herpes, fetal scalp monitors should be used only when absolutely necessary. An alternative is the external monitor, which tracks the baby's heartbeat through the mother's abdomen. This isn't sufficient in all situations, but it carries no risk.

Lastly, while women with genital HSV-1 have fewer outbreaks and less shedding, they are still at risk of transmitting the virus to the baby at birth, so the information in this section may be important to them as well.

PREVENTION: MEN WITH RECURRENT HERPES

As we've seen, the risk of neonatal herpes is highest when the expectant mother first becomes infected with HSV during late pregnancy. Men can play a critical role in minimizing this risk in some situations. For example, let's look at a common scenario: Phil and Carla have been married for two years, and Carla is now pregnant for the first time. Phil has had herpes for eight years. They don't have sex when he's having an outbreak, and so far she seems not to have been infected. But what if she gets infected with herpes for the first time during pregnancy? This is a very high-risk situation, especially in the last trimester. What should they do?

First, let's remember that most people who are infected with HSV-2 don't know it, and this might include Carla. Considering the fact of her exposure, she should be tested with a type-specific HSV serology to determine whether she truly is uninfected.

If type-specific serology confirms that Carla is not infected with HSV, she and Phil should, at a minimum, refrain from all sexual activity during pregnancy when Phil is symptomatic, and should also use condoms for sex between outbreaks. In addition, Phil may choose to take antiviral medication suppressively to lower his rate of asymptomatic shedding and potentially reduce the likelihood of transmission. Perhaps most important, many experts recommend abstaining from sex altogether as a sensible precaution during the third trimester. Remember that a substantial number of neonatal herpes cases are caused by HSV-1. So if Phil has a history of cold sores, avoiding oral-genital contact should also be part of the prevention plan.

Whatever precautions the couple chooses to take or not take, it's important that Carla's doctor or midwife be informed that Phil has herpes and she doesn't.

In this example, of course, Phil knew he had herpes and disclosed it to Carla. Yet as we have discussed throughout the book, many millions of men are not aware they have genital herpes but are capable of transmitting it all the same. Because of this, some experts advocate routine serologic testing of all pregnant women. The purpose of this is to identify women who are *not* infected and therefore at risk of acquiring HSV during pregnancy, with all the risks to the baby that this implies. Serologic testing is not done routinely as yet, but it is being debated in the health policy arena.

WHEN NEWBORNS GET HERPES

Many babies are exposed to small amounts of HSV at birth yet resist infection, and all of the precautions outlined above are helpful in reducing the risk. But some babies are infected with HSV at birth, and the consequences can often be severe. For infants, herpes is not just the possibility of an irritating rash. HSV can overpower the immature immune system. Without timely diagnosis and antiviral therapy over half of infected babies die and about half of the survivors have lasting brain damage.

Babies rarely show signs of herpes at birth. Neonatal infection—even in very serious cases—may cause no sores on the skin at all. Typically, however, herpes symptoms develop within several days to three weeks. These can include the classic herpes lesions seen in adults as well as convulsions, jaundice, pneumonia, fussiness, fever, red swollen eyes (conjunctivitis), and lack of interest in food.

Because the initial symptoms of neonatal herpes infection overlap with those of more common newborn illnesses, diagnosis can be quite difficult. Viral culture is often used as a diagnostic test. Recently, a more sensitive DNA test called *polymerase chain reaction* (PCR) has been used to diagnose HSV infection and now is recommended in this setting.

The severity of herpes in newborns varies greatly. If infection is confined to the skin, eyes, and mouth, the infant's prognosis is usually good. But sometimes in newborns the virus can infect the blood and spread widely. In another frequent complication, herpes can attack the brain (encephalitis), often causing irreversible damage.

With any form of neonatal infection, early diagnosis and treatment are critical. Acyclovir is effective in many cases. Many doctors will start an infant on acyclovir even before a herpes diagnosis is confirmed, provided there is strong suspicion that HSV is the cause of the infant's illness. Some doctors also will treat an infant if the mother was having a first episode of HSV infection during vaginal delivery, because the chances of transmission in this situation are so high.

PROTECTING THE BABY AT HOME

Even when a baby is born without herpes, it's important to remember there is still a risk of infection, and herpes can be a very serious illness in the first few weeks of life. Mothers and fathers with active herpes sores should take care to protect their babies. If you're having an outbreak (or even if you're not), some logical precautions include the following:

• Wash your hands before touching the baby.

• *If you have cold sores on your mouth,* wear a mask when you handle the baby to keep from inadvertently touching your mouth and then the baby.

• *If a visiting friend or relative has a cold sore,* warn him or her about the risks of spreading HSV to your newborn through a kiss or through careless touching and ask that he or she visit when the cold sores resolves.

The point here is not to discourage all the touching and cuddling that go along with taking care of a newborn. That kind of contact is very necessary. But if you're having an outbreak, or a relative or friend is having an outbreak, safety is an important concern, and you'll want to take steps to protect your child.

NEONATAL HERPES AND ADVOCACY

People with HSV are not generally organized in a lobby for changes in health policy, but neonatal herpes is one area in which the need for advocacy has begun to present itself. While the risk of neonatal herpes may be small in any individual pregnancy, the total number of new cases per year—now estimated at between 400 and 2800—is high enough to warrant a concerted prevention program. With many other diseases and conditions, including several STIs, medical guidelines dictate routine screening in pregnancy or interventions around the time of delivery to protect mother and baby. A number of herpes experts joined together in 2005 to publish a journal article calling on the CDC to make neonatal herpes a reportable disease, so that the nation would have more reliable data upon which to base future prevention programs. They point out that routine testing is done in pregnancy for rubella, gonorrhea, syphilis, and HIV infection, and not a single one of these has an annual incidence that reaches even the lowest estimate of neonatal herpes. Perhaps in future years this movement will galvanize additional support to mobilize funding for research on which types of interventions can truly lower the risk of neonatal herpes further.

WHAT YOU CAN DO

Many of the decisions about managing herpes at delivery call for discussion with your doctor or midwife. Be sure to tell your healthcare provider about your (or your partner's) history of genital herpes. Ask the provider to tell you about his or her standard procedures and the hospital's procedures regarding herpes, pregnancy, and delivery. Some of the questions you should ask are:

• How does your doctor or midwife determine the need for a C-section?

• Will he or she perform a thorough visual exam looking for

signs of genital herpes early in labor?

• What types of monitors are routinely used? When might a fetal scalp monitor be used?

You also need to tell your obstetric healthcare provider if you plan to take (or have already taken) an antiviral drug during pregnancy. And of course, you'll want to tell your provider if you experience symptoms of herpes just prior to labor.

While it's smart to make plans in case you do have a herpes outbreak, keep in mind that the vast majority of women will not have an outbreak at delivery. And, as we've stressed, if you have a history of recurrent genital herpes, your baby already possesses antibodies to the virus. It's the babies born to mothers having a first episode during pregnancy who are at the highest risk of getting sick. Either way, it's important to be proactive about prevention.

15

THE BROADER SPECTRUM OF HSV INFECTION

In putting together this book, we've placed great emphasis on the fact that genital herpes is a very common infection that is certainly manageable—and for some people altogether trivial. We want people to keep herpes in this perspective.

You may, however, hear or read statements about herpes simplex that alarm you. Some may fall into the category of "herpes myths"— pure misinformation, such as the idea that people with herpes should never donate blood. Other statements, however, may prove to be accurate information that relates to *rare types* of HSV infection.

In reviewing what experts call the "full clinical spectrum" of HSV infection, we find a number of uncommon conditions that can result when either HSV-1 or HSV-2 breaks out of its usual pattern of latency and minor reactivations. In describing these conditions here, we run the risk of scaring you with what may sound like irrelevant information. If we were creating a book for drivers' education, this would be like including a whole chapter on what to do if all four tires go flat at once. Nonetheless, we do want this book to serve as a useful information resource. We think it's important, therefore, to establish some basic facts about herpes complications, and to quash some of the misinformation currently spread.

HERPETIC WHITLOW

Among the forms of autoinoculation (self infection) already mentioned, herpetic whitlow, a herpes infection of the fingertip, deserves further explanation because it can occur in a number of ways. Generally, whitlow results when virus is spread to a finger that has a cut or to the softer tissue of the nail cuticle. Once there, it can cause an outbreak with symptoms similar to those of oral-facial or genital herpes. Herpetic whitlow can also recur.

First, of course, the virus has to get to the finger. In people who have genital herpes, this is most likely to occur from touching your own lesions during a first episode (as was explained in Chapter 4). However, not all cases of whitlow result from genital herpes infection. Some cases have been traced to adults who have an HSV-1 infection on the mouth or face and are in the habit of biting their fingernails. An active HSV-1 infection can deposit virus in saliva, and nail biting can create an opening in the skin that allows HSV a portal of entry.

In the past, herpetic whitlow afflicted significant numbers of dentists, respiratory therapists, and other healthcare professionals whose hands were frequently in contact with patients' saliva. In recent years, however, the widespread use of latex gloves appears to have reduced the incidence of whitlow among healthcare workers.

Today, most whitlow is caused by HSV-2 in sexually active adults, almost always the result of hand contact with lesions during a first episode of genital herpes, prior to the development of a full immune response. Though the risk of herpetic whitlow is small in those with recurrent genital herpes, it's a good idea to avoid touching HSV lesions. If you do make contact, wash your hands right away.

Soap and water will kill the virus and avert the risk of whitlow. And if you have oral-facial herpes, remember that biting your nails can be risky.

OCULAR HERPES

Ocular herpes, meaning HSV infection of the eye, is almost always caused by HSV-1 in adults and children. In newborn babies, it can be caused by HSV-2 acquired from the mother during birth. Ocular herpes usually occurs when latent HSV-1 from an earlier infection in the facial area reactivates and travels to the eye instead of the mouth or lips, but the eye can also be the site of a first infection. Less than 5% of people with an oral HSV-1 infection develop ocular herpes.

Symptoms sometimes begin with blisters or cold sores on the eyelid and the itchy, watery sort of "pink eye" associated with conjunctivitis. Later symptoms typically include pain and sensitivity to light. Left untreated, ocular herpes can lead to painful lesions on the cornea. Anyone with suspected herpes infection of the eye should seek evaluation by a specialist. Various kinds of eyedrops can be used, depending on the nature of the infection and which layers of the cornea may be affected. Some of these treatments are topical antivirals, such as trifluridine, acyclovir, and vidarabine. Treatment options also include oral antivirals and, in some cases, steroidal eyedrops.

More than 25% of people with ocular herpes experience recurrences. Repeated recurrences can result in corneal scarring, overgrowth of new blood vessels in the eye, and permanent corneal scarring that may necessitate transplantation to restore vision. However, proper medical care can help to avert these complications.

HSV INFECTIONS OF THE NERVOUS SYSTEM

HSV can cause an infection of the nervous system called *meningitis*. Meningitis is an inflammation of the meninges, the protective membranes that cover the brain and spinal cord, and can be caused by a number of different infectious agents. When the cause is bacterial, the infection is called *septic meningitis*; when the cause is viral, it's called *aseptic meningitis*.

In adults, most cases of meningitis occur as a complication of a first infection with HSV-2. HSV meningitis is seen in more than 30% of women and about 10% of men experiencing a first HSV-2 infection. The principal symptoms include fever, stiff neck, intense headache, and aversion to bright light. Fortunately, HSV meningitis generally clears up by itself, recurs only infrequently, and causes no damage to the central nervous system. However, symptoms of numbness, tingling, muscle weakness, and difficult urination that are sometimes present with HSV meningitis may persist for a few months. Recurrence can be expected in 20% to 30% of cases, usually in association with a reactivation of genital herpes, but recurrent episodes of HSV meningitis tend to be milder than first episodes.

HSV is also linked to an extremely serious though extremely rare infection called *encephalitis*, which is an infection of the brain tissue itself. In adults, HSV encephalitis is almost always caused by HSV-1. In newborns, either HSV-1 or HSV-2 can cause encephalitis. One reason it's so critical to prevent HSV infection in newborns is that they are much more susceptible to encephalitis because of their immature immune system. (See Chapter 14 for more information on neonatal HSV infection and its prevention.)

Among adults, about half the cases of HSV encephalitis are first infections of HSV-1, while the rest occur as a complication of recur-

THE BROADER SPECTRUM OF HSV INFECTION

rent infection. In either case, course and outcome are the same. HSV encephalitis is marked initially by fever, headache, and confusion, but patients rapidly suffer more serious effects such as seizure and delirium. Only about 1,000 cases are seen each year in the U.S., but without antiviral therapy, 70% of those afflicted will die. Survivors may suffer permanent brain damage.

DISSEMINATED HSV INFECTION AND HSV INFECTION IN THE IMMUNOCOMPROMISED

Viremia refers to the presence of virus in the bloodstream. Viremia is probably present to some extent in every case of primary (first) infection with HSV, but in otherwise healthy individuals with normal immune function, it's usually not a problem. It is possible, however, for HSV in the bloodstream to cause a widespread HSV infection called a *disseminated* infection, which may cause extensive lesions on the skin and affect internal organs as well. (Even in cases that appear to be limited to the skin, some internal lesions are likely.) Disseminated HSV infection is a serious condition that requires immediate medical attention and antiviral therapy. A number of organs may be involved, but the liver is the focus of greatest concern.

Those most susceptible to disseminated HSV infection are people whose immune systems are suppressed *(or compromised)*. Immunocompromise can occur naturally as a congenital defect, or it can be induced by malnutrition, severe burn injury, diseases such as HIV/AIDS and cancer, radical medical interventions such as radiation therapy, or immunosuppressive drugs used to prevent rejection of transplanted organs and tissues.

People with suppressed immune systems are sometimes vulnerable to complications if they have either genital or oral-facial HSV.

Some with recurrent genital herpes have lengthy outbreaks that must be treated with antiviral medication. People with AIDS, in particular, may have severe and lengthy outbreaks. In fact, HSV is one of the so-called *opportunistic infections* that define a patient's transition from being merely HIV-positive to having AIDS.

Acyclovir, valacyclovir, and famciclovir are often used to treat HSV infection in AIDS patients. Episodic or suppressive therapeutic strategies may be followed, but in either case, the patient often receives doses higher than those given to patients with normal immune function. Even at higher doses, first-line antiviral therapy may fail to control the infection

While the interaction between HSV and HIV has many facets, a major reason for treatment failure is the emergence of virus that is resistant or less sensitive to acyclovir or penciclovir. Naturally occurring resistant strains of HSV are found in about 1% of people with normal immune function, but even so, these strains are of no known clinical significance, as most patients respond to antiviral therapy regardless of the presence of resistant strains. In immunocompromised patients, however, HSV (including resistant strains) is present in much greater volume. Antiviral therapy knocks out the susceptible strains, but the patient's lack of natural defenses and the presence of an unusually large amount of resistant virus can lead to the overgrowth of resistant virus and a persistent infection that is immune to first-line antiviral therapy. In these cases, clinicians will often use medications such as intravenous foscarnet or the topical drugs cidofovir, trifluridine, or imiquimod, which have a different way of attacking HSV.

The emergence of resistant strains of bacteria due to the overuse and misuse of antibiotics has become a very real problem, especially in the hospital setting. Clinicians have naturally been concerned that the widespread use of acyclovir might also lead to the emergence of resistant HSV, which could be problematic for the general immunocompetent population. But so far, no evidence has been found to suggest that this concern is warranted.

HSV INFECTION AND BLOOD DONATION

ASHA has occasionally fielded questions and comments from people who have been deferred from donating blood because they had a recurring herpes infection or because they were on daily suppressive antiviral therapy. According to the national office of the American Red Cross, neither daily antiviral therapy nor recurrent HSV infection itself are legitimate grounds for deferral. At a national level, the Red Cross policy recognizes that HSV resides primarily in the nervous system, not in the blood, and there is no documented case of HSV transmission via blood infusion. However, it is clear from the occasional calls to ASHA that local chapters of the Red Cross may have varying interpretations—or misinterpretations—of the rules and regulations.

As noted earlier in this chapter, some degree of HSV viremia (HSV in the bloodstream) is probably present in the majority of first infections. While this HSV viremia is of no known relevance when it comes to blood donation, it is advisable to abstain from blood donation during a first episode of HSV infection. Aside from the fact that you may have at least some small amount of HSV in your bloodstream, it's also true that you're unwell just now. Chances are if you are in the midst of a true first HSV infection, donating blood is the last thing you'll feel like doing, and it just doesn't make sense to further weaken yourself by giving blood. In fact, donating blood is not recommended for persons with flu or any other acute illness.

And even though there are no official blood-donation restrictions for persons subject to recurrent HSV infection, if you are having a recurrence and feeling sick with the symptoms, it makes more sense to wait until the current outbreak subsides.

THE BOTTOM LINE

If you have genital herpes, take precautions to avoid the problems of autoinoculation. If you experience a first episode of HSV infection, avoid touching the lesions, and wash your hands immediately afterward if you do touch them. This simple step can help you avoid herpetic whitlow. Also, remember to keep your hands away from your eyes when HSV is active. Most cases of ocular herpes in adults are due to HSV-1, but it is possible to transfer HSV-2 by hand from genital lesions to your eyes.

Remember that complications such as disseminated HSV infection are most likely to appear in people with compromised immune systems. If you have a history of herpes infection and are to undergo cancer treatment (or any other procedure or intervention) that could suppress your immune function, tell your doctor about your medical history so prophylactic antiviral therapy can be considered. The same advice goes for people who are newly diagnosed with HIV: Tell your doctor if you have a history of herpes infection. You may benefit from suppressive antiviral therapy.

16

DIAGNOSTIC TESTS

"Two years ago I had some sores on my labia and went to the doctor," says a caller to the National Herpes Hotline. "He just looked at them and told me I had herpes. Then he gave me a prescription and said I might have more trouble later on. Well, I haven't had any symptoms in all this time, and I'm wondering: maybe this isn't herpes. Could it be something else?"

Herpes simplex is the most common cause of genital sores or ulcers in the United States, and often it can be recognized by the trained eye of a medical professional. However, HSV can be confused with other infections, and some people have good reason to question the diagnosis they received. In one recent study, the rate of false positive diagnosis was 20%, and other studies have pointed to an even greater likelihood of false negatives—meaning that herpes is more often underdiagnosed. Consequently, we recommend that everyone who visits a doctor for treatment of herpes request a laboratory test; this can confirm a diagnosis that may have been based on visual clues or the patient's medical history.

VIRAL CULTURE

There are several diagnostic tests currently available, and more reach the market each year. When a lesion is present, the test still used most often to diagnose herpes is called *viral culture*. Using a swab, the healthcare provider gathers infected cells from an active herpes lesion. The swab is then placed into a special solution and sent to a laboratory. At the lab, virus from the swab is allowed to grow for several days in a collection of healthy cells. If HSV is indeed present on the swab, it will cause certain changes in the cell culture that can be seen under a microscope. In essence, viral culture transplants the virus into another setting and allows it to grow until its effects on cells are visible. Then the cells can be stained with a specific antibody that will react with one or both HSV types to confirm that the virus is herpes simplex.

The major advantage of viral culture is its *specificity,* meaning it will not be positive for herpes simplex virus if another infection is causing the cell changes.

Though viral culture is the most widely used laboratory test for HSV, it does have drawbacks and limitations. Samples for viral culture must be taken when and where virus can be found, either from lesions on the surface of the skin or from mucous membranes on internal surfaces, such as those of the cervix. The best samples come from lesions that contain large amounts of virus and have not yet had a chance to form a crust or scab. If the target lesion is in the process of healing, viral culture often yields a false negative result: The swab doesn't pick up enough live virus, and the test fails to find HSV, even though herpes really is the culprit. Viral culture is most likely to be positive (80% to 90% of the time) during first episodes, when large amounts of virus are present. During recurrent episodes, the likelihood of a positive result is only around 30%. In technical terms, then, while culture has good specificity, it is not highly sensitive.

Another potential disadvantage of viral culture is that it often takes many hours before cellular changes occur in the culture medium, so the results are anything but rapid. Most lab reports take from two to seven days for completion, and waiting for the results may test your patience. Though clearly not infallible, viral culture remains the most widely used tool for an initial herpes diagnosis, if lesions are present.

Viral culture costs anywhere from $40 to $120 (depending on the lab chosen and not including the cost of an office visit). If the results are negative and your healthcare provider has good reason to suspect HSV anyway, you should arrange to come back to the office promptly the next time you have an outbreak so a better sample can be obtained.

PCR TESTING

Polymerase chain reaction, or PCR, is a type of test you may begin hearing more about as an alternative to viral culture for diagnosis when lesions are present. As with culture, this test detects virus that has reactivated and traveled from the nerves to the skin—genital skin, for example. Samples can be taken with a swab. More sensitive than viral culture or any of the other technologies listed here, PCR offers a very rapid, extremely sensitive, type-specific diagnostic test for HSV. It's currently used for clinical diagnosis by many of the country's top university laboratories, and some commercial laboratories now have it on the market. In particular, PCR has become the test of choice for herpes infections of the central nervous system (meningitis and encephalitis) and HSV infection in newborns. While viral culture remains the test most often used, PCR seems likely to replace culture for suspected HSV lesions in the next decade as its availability increases.

TYPE 1 OR TYPE 2?

As we've already said, it's useful to know whether your herpes symptoms are caused by HSV-1 or HSV-2, the major reason being that genital HSV-1 infection is less likely to cause frequent recurrent outbreaks. If you're in the midst of a first episode, you might find it reassuring to know you're dealing with the less troublesome of the two viral types. Determining viral type can be done in a number of ways. Most commonly, lab technicians take an HSV sample grown in cell culture—a proven HSV specimen—and expose it to type-specific antibodies. As mentioned above, viral typing is often a routine step for confirming the cell changes in HSV cultures, entailing no additional costs. To be certain about this, however, if your clinician takes a viral culture for HSV, you may want to ask that if the virus grows, the type should be identified.

TYPE-SPECIFIC SEROLOGY

One of the disadvantages of all the viral culture methods and the confirmatory tests described above is that they only work well when herpes is in its active phase and genital sores are present. But what about the person who has had only one outbreak and now questions the diagnosis? What about all the people who have mild symptoms that test negative in a viral culture, or those whose partners develop herpes and claim they have not been unfaithful? Perhaps more important, what about all the people who are infected with HSV but are unaware of it?

One diagnostic tool that skirts the problem of sampling active lesions is a blood test called a *serologic assay* or, more simply, a *serology*. HSV serologic assays detect antibodies to HSV that are made by your body as a natural defensive response to infection. Immune response varies from one individual to the next, so it's difficult to say exactly how long it may take for detectable antibodies to form. However, beginning just a few days after initial infection with HSV, antibodies are produced in growing numbers. Within a few weeks to a few months, they can be detected by serologic tests, whether HSV is in an active phase or not. Their presence certifies infection. Thus, serologic tests are a standard method of diagnosing a number of infections that a person may have acquired in the past. For example, the standard HIV test is a serologic test for antibodies to HIV.

A serologic assay can be a powerful diagnostic tool, but only if it can tell the difference between HSV-1 and HSV-2 infections. Here's the problem: More than half of adults in the U.S. are infected with HSV-1 (the "cold sore" virus, usually acquired in childhood). If the serology used is not *type-specific* (that is, able to distinguish HSV-1 antibodies from HSV-2 antibodies), a positive result really tells us nothing about the likelihood of genital herpes. The test may just be detecting an earlier oral HSV-1 infection and is, therefore, effectively worthless. Unfortunately, many serologies claim to be type-specific, with lab reports that purport to show separate readings for HSV-1 and HSV-2, but actually cross-react with antibodies for either viral type (and sometimes with other herpesviruses). What shows up as HSV-2 may really be HSV-1 and vice versa. In fact, many experts believe these nonspecific serologic tests should be taken off the market or clearly labeled as unable to distinguish between antibodies to HSV-1 and HSV-2.

Does this mean it's best to write off serologies altogether? No. In today's marketplace, bona fide serologic tests that are truly type-specific can be easily located. With these tests, patients can know for certain what researchers call their *serostatus*—that is, do they have HSV-1, HSV-2, neither, or both? And patients can know this whether they have symptomatic outbreaks or not. These type-specific serologic tests have proved extremely valuable in research to determine the extent of herpes infection among adults and in the study of patterns of viral shedding and other aspects of how HSV behaves in the body. In a wide range of research studies, type-specific serology is a valuable tool for understanding the intricacies of HSV.

Serologic testing has changed rapidly in recent years and is no longer confined to the research setting. As of this writing there are a number of commercially available tests, which are named by brand here to minimize confusion. *(See HSV Diagnostic Tests: Performance Characteristics, next page.)* Focus Diagnostics manufactures two different type-specific serologic tests that can be used for HSV, both of which are branded HerpeSelect®. These are now routinely available through Quest Diagnostics, one of the two largest providers of medical laboratory services in the United States. The HerpeSelect® tests, both of which require a standard blood draw, require one to two weeks for results. They have been studied in various populations and have been in clinical use for eight years, following FDA approval in 1999.

Also approved in 1999 was a point-of-care test for HSV-2 that can be done with a serum sample from a finger prick. Assuming the provider has the proper lab facilities, results are available in less than 10 minutes. This product was launched as the POCkit HSV-2 Rapid Test but is now marketed as the **biokit**HSV-2 Rapid Test or Sure-Vue™ HSV-2 Rapid Test.

The assays by Focus Diagnostics and biokit USA are well-known

HSV DIAGNOSTIC TESTS: PERFORMANCE CHARACTERISTICS

TYPE-SPECIFIC SEROLOGIC TESTS				
Test	Source	Sensitivity	Specificity	Comments
HerpeSelect® 1&2 ELISA	Focus Diagnostics, Inc. www.herpeselect.com or call 1-800-838-4548	96-100% (HSV-2) 91-96% (HSV-1)	96-100% (HSV-2) 92-100% (HSV-1)	Blood draw, best for hi-volume labs. Results in 1 to 2 weeks.
HerpeSelect® 1&2 Immunoblot	Focus Diagnostics, Inc. www.herpeselect.com or call 1-800-838-4548	97-100% (HSV-2) 99-100% (HSV-1)	94-98% (HSV-2) 93-100% (HSV-1)	Blood draw, best for lo-volume labs. Results in 1 to 2 weeks.
biokitHSV-2 Rapid Test	biokit USA www.biokitusa.com or call 1-800-926-3353	77-100% (HSV-2)†	71-98% (HSV-2)†	Finger prick or blood draw, results in 10 minutes. Sensitivity and specificity affected by reading variability. Also available from Fisher HealthCare as the Sure-Vue™ HSV-2 Rapid Test.
CAPTIA™ HSV IgG type-specific ELISA	Trinity Biotech USA www.trinitybiotech.com or call 1-800-325-3424	97-100% (HSV-2) 88% (HSV-1)	90-92% (HSV-2) 98-100% (HSV-1)	Blood draw.
Western blot assay	Available only through U. Washington http://dcpts/washington.edu/rspvirus/ or call 1-800-713-5198	>97%†	>98%‡	Blood draw, gold standard for TSST, no commercial distribution. Requires 1-2 weeks. Results are mailed or faxed to healthcare provider.

SOURCE: *Herpes Testing Toolkit*, American Social Health Association, Inc. © Copyright 2006.

Sensitivity and specificity ranges for serologic tests come from package inserts/FDA approvals of each test for performance characteristics in sexually active adults and pregnant women. The HerpeSelect® and Western blot assays have an established performance history. Numbers for **biokit**HSV-2 Rapid Test reflect also highest and lowest values as reported in package inserts. However, subsequent studies have posted values in the 90s for sensitivity and specificity.

and inspire confidence among researchers in this field, but there are also relative newcomers, such as the CAPTIA™ HSV IgG type-specific ELISA by Trinity Biotech USA. Kits by other manufacturers may join these in the commercial market, pending FDA approval. Another point-of-care test, tentatively called Express, is currently in development by Focus and is expected to be available by late 2007 or early 2008.

The "gold standard" of HSV serologic testing is the Western blot, developed by academic research labs such as the Virology Laboratory at the University of Washington in Seattle. This test has been used in many research studies and is available from the University of Washington by request to private practitioners around the United States. (See Table on page 179 for additional information.)

It's also important to mention that HerpeSelect® is by far the most commonly used serologic test, and because of this we know more about how well it works. One key finding is that people whose tests have a low-positive reading on the HerpeSelect® pt HSV-2 ELISA—a reading between 1.1 and 3.5—have only a 50% chance of being HSV-2-positive as measured by other tests. Such persons have so-called 'indeterminate results," and these tests should be confirmed by a second test using another method, such as HSV Western Blot or biokit.

Some individuals infected with HSV-2 will develop antibodies that can be detected by these type-specific tests within two weeks, but most will not. For this reason, experts usually recommend that patients wait twelve to sixteen weeks after exposure to HSV before seeking a serologic test.

As valuable as type-specific serology has proved to be, there are practical limits to its usefulness. It's important that you understand exactly what a serologic result means:

- If your serologic test is positive for HSV-2, we know that you have been infected with HSV-2 at some time in the past (but we don't know when). You should assume that your HSV-2 infection is a genital infection for the simple reason that almost all HSV-2 infections are genital. This is true even if you've never experienced any genital symptoms.

- If your serology is positive for HSV-1, we know that you have been infected with HSV-1 at some time in your life, and while it is probably an oral-facial infection (even if you have no history of cold sores), you should be aware that a growing number of genital herpes infections are caused by HSV 1.

- If your test result is negative for HSV-1 and HSV-2, you're not out of the woods just yet. Remember, type-specific serologies detect antibodies to HSV and are of limited value during and immediately after a first episode of infection, because you may not have had adequate time to form antibodies to the virus.

Type-specific serology can be of tremendous value in a number of settings. Remember Phil and Carla, the expectant parents in Chapter 14? Phil knew he had genital herpes; Carla's serostatus was unknown but presumed to be negative. If it truly were the case that Carla had never been infected with HSV-1 or HSV-2 and thus had no antibodies to either virus, an accurate type-specific serology could alert Carla's obstetric caregivers to a potentially serious complication; namely, that of Carla's acquiring a first HSV infection late in her pregnancy, a dangerous circumstance for the newborn.

Type-specific serology is also valuable in cases where a patient has reason to question a herpes diagnosis that was never confirmed by laboratory test. Take the case of Larry, who was given a visual diagnosis of herpes years ago but whose viral culture always came back negative. He has only the mildest rash in the genital area about once a year. Is this really herpes? Taken together with his history, a serology positive for HSV-2 is strong evidence that the answer is yes.

Type-specific serology can also simplify a couple's sex life and relieve the stress and apprehension of HSV transmission. Imagine a case in which one partner in the couple (let's call them Cathy and Rich) has a confirmed HSV-2 infection, and the other partner's serostatus is unknown. Cathy knows she has genital herpes, and Rich *thinks* he does not. Rich could undergo a type-specific serologic test, and if the result came back positive for HSV-2, the couple could quit worrying about Rich acquiring genital herpes from Cathy. They might then choose to forego precautions such as condom use or daily suppressive therapy, if concern about HSV transmission were the reason motivating either of these actions.

As this technology hits the market, the biggest problem for patients and healthcare providers alike may be distinguishing the quality tests from the impostors. Guidelines published by the American Medical Association, the U.S. Centers for Disease Control and Prevention, and the California Department of Health Services are intended to help medical professionals sort through the conflicting claims of diagnostic companies and identify the truly accurate serologic tests. In 2004 and again in 2006, ASHA published a *Herpes Testing Toolkit,* which discusses these tests and their potential uses for a clinical audience. Readers wishing to get more information on herpes testing can go to the ASHA Web site at www.ASHAstd.org

or contact the STI Resource Center. (See Resource List on page 221 for Web site and telephone listings for the diagnostic tests mentioned above.)

DEBATE OVER USES FOR TYPE-SPECIFIC SEROLOGY

In addition to possible confusion over which tests are the most accurate, there is also some disagreement among medical experts as to the best uses for type-specific blood tests. In which situations should they be employed? Can they be relied upon for diagnosing a person with an apparent first episode? Will they have value in testing someone who has a history of unexplained genital symptoms? Should they be used in testing all persons at risk for herpes?

While these and other questions are still under discussion, there is emerging consensus that type-specific serologic tests will be very helpful in several clinical situations:

• **History of recurrent genital symptoms:** In many cases, patients present to a healthcare provider seeking diagnosis of genital symptoms that recur from time to time but are not present at the time of the clinic visit. When the patient's history (including risk factors and description of symptoms) suggests the possibility of herpes, a serologic test can provide very useful information. Specifically, a test result positive for HSV-2 would be a very strong indication that herpes had been causing the symptoms.

• **Discordant couples:** If one partner has been diagnosed with herpes and the couple is faced with decisions about how to prevent the spread of genital herpes, the first question demanding an answer might be this: Does the second partner already have herpes anyway? As we showed in the early chapters of this book, it's quite common for an individual to have herpes and not know it. Testing may provide the information that both partners already have the same serotype, and this would mean they faced little or no risk of transmission anyway.

• **Confirmation of clinical diagnosis:** If a patient was diagnosed through a visual examination or a culture that was not typed, confirming and typing genital herpes infections through type-specific serology can aid in prognostic, medication, and prevention decisions, as the clinical outcomes for HSV-2 and HSV-1 genital infections are quite different. Similarly, type-specific tests can be used sometimes in situations where a patient has a genital lesion but direct viral detection (culture, PCR, antigen detection) proves to be problematic or is negative.

In addition to these scenarios, type-specific serologic tests have been utilized in a variety of other situations, including routine HSV testing in HIV and other immunocompromised patients, in patients at high risk of HIV, and in sexual assault cases. Perhaps most hotly debated have been the following two potential uses of HSV serologic tests:

• **STI screening:** Many people have reason to seek a medical check-up to find out whether they are free of sexually transmitted infections. Perhaps, for example, they have a relatively new partner, have initially used condoms as a precaution, and now are reconsidering the question of whether any form of safe sex is really necessary. A visit to the healthcare provider, they reason, will provide a thorough check for STIs.

First of all, it should be mentioned that there is a wide range of practices when it comes to STI testing, and even some common infections such as chlamydia may not be part of a clinician's routine testing. And before the advent of commercial serologic tests for HSV, there was really no practical way of testing for herpes unless genital lesions were present. Now that serologic tests are widely available, the question becomes: Should these tests be more widely used? Experts take a variety of positions on this, but a growing number support the idea that a person requesting to be "checked for STIs" should be offered an HSV serologic test—or, at the very least, should be informed (if the test is not routinely available) that they are *not* being tested for herpes when they request their STI checkup. The public health community is slowly adopting this approach.

- **Routine testing of pregnant women:** As we explained in Chapter 14, the risk of neonatal herpes is highest when a pregnant woman acquires genital herpes during pregnancy. The role of serologic testing, then, would be to identify women who are free of HSV infection—who are at risk for either HSV-1 or HSV-2. Once identified, these sero-negative women could be made aware of the risk of acquiring herpes from a sexual partner and could be educated about prevention measures such as use of condoms or abstaining from sex in the third trimester. A number of experts in this area have suggested a model in which serologic tests can also be offered to the partners of sero-negative women, to determine whether a risk of transmission exists within that particular couple. In any case where a pregnant woman is sero-negative and her partner is positive for genital herpes, use of suppressive antiviral therapy by the partner might be another strategy to decrease the risk of transmission.

The notion of routine blood testing for women in pregnancy poses a number of challenges, as mentioned in Chapter 14, and as of this writing there are no published guidelines for the use of such an approach.

OTHER COMMON DIAGNOSTIC TOOLS

Apart from the fast-growing interest in PCR, the alternatives to the viral culture and type-specific serology are few. Antigen tests can be employed when lesions are present, with a sample taken using a swab. In terms of accuracy and cost, these assays are generally comparable to viral culture, but they are seldom used any more.

Other testing methods sometimes used to diagnose herpes include the Tzanck test and Pap test to identify HSV-infected cells. A physician scrapes herpes lesions and may treat the sample with various stains. When the samples are examined under a microscope, certain telltale signs of herpes infection can be spotted by the trained eye. These procedures are rapid and simple, but they require a "judgment call" by the lab technician. Under a microscope, changes caused by other herpesviruses may look very similar to those caused by HSV, so both tests leave lots of room for human error.

An additional word about Pap tests is in order. Many women

believe that their annual or biannual Pap test looks for a number of STIs and that a normal result indicates the absence of STIs. Unfortunately, this is not true. Pap tests check for abnormal cells in cervical tissue, and by proxy, often detect an STI called human papillomavirus. But a Pap test is not a specific test for any STI and is not used to look for HSV. However, occasionally a Pap test will detect cell changes that look like those caused by HSV.

17

NEW RESEARCH, NEW HOPE

Living in a world of rapid scientific and technological change, we'd like to think that any day now modern medicine will find a way to wipe out genital herpes instead of just holding it in check. But the truth is, we're unlikely to see a real cure any time soon.

The great difficulty in developing a cure lies in the dual nature of herpes simplex virus infection—it has active *and* latent phases. Today's antiviral drugs (acyclovir, valacyclovir, and famciclovir) are very effective against *active* virus, such as HSV replicating in the skin. In fact, these antivirals are effectively "switched on" by an enzyme that is produced only when HSV is replicating (active). But today's antivirals do nothing to combat dormant HSV, because dormant HSV doesn't put out the requisite chemical signals.

Further complicating the challenge is the fact that any drug developed to root out latent HSV infection must locate and eliminate dormant virus without killing the nerve cells (ganglia) in which it resides. Nerve tissue poses an especially tricky problem because it doesn't regenerate; kill too many nerve cells, and the cure is worse than the disease.

Does all this mean there's no hope? Has medical science given up? No—not by a long shot. In the five years since the last edition of this book, we have seen the findings from the valacyclovir transmission study, which proved the concept that suppressive therapy reduces risk of transmission, and we have seen the start of a final-phase clinical trial for a herpes vaccine that may provide partial protection in women. We have not seen major breakthroughs that promise dramatically new therapies or vaccines in the short term, but much work is being done, and some of it may bear fruit. We will review some of the more prominent research here.

VACCINE RESEARCH AND DEVELOPMENT

Just about everyone in this country has some experience with vaccination. Tens of millions of Americans have a small round scar on their upper arm where they were vaccinated for smallpox during childhood. Most of us have been vaccinated for hepatitis, polio, tetanus, and a host of other infectious diseases.

Vaccination introduces a foreign substance (an antigen) into our bodies in a controlled manner, so our immune system has a chance to prepare a response to the antigen. This response includes the body's production of antibodies as well as the cellular immune response described in Chapter 4. Both of these internal defense systems fight off infection when we are exposed to disease-causing bacteria and viruses. The idea is that vaccination will cause production of sufficient antibodies, or a sufficiently strong cellular immune response, to ward off future infection.

While all vaccines attempt to enhance immunity, some are designed to be delivered *prior* to exposure to a given pathogen, while others may be given *after* infection has occurred. The first category is sometimes referred to by the term *prophylactic vaccine*. With these, the desired outcome may be to prevent infection altogether—what could be called "sterilizing immunity." On the other hand, a prophylactic vaccine may be brought to market with the less ambitious but important expectation that it will provide partial immunity. In this scenario, the microbe may be able to replicate within the human, but because the host is prepared to make antibodies or T cells to attack a specific pathogen, the symptoms of the infection are markedly reduced, and the public health is advanced because the infection is much less likely to be transmitted.

With the second broad category, *therapeutic vaccine*, the vaccine is delivered to a person who is already known to be infected with a particular pathogen. Here again, the benefit may be reducing symptoms—and also, possibly, limiting contagiousness.

With regard to HSV infection, researchers are exploring both ways to use vaccines: Prophylactically, to prevent HSV-2 infection from becoming established; and therapeutically, to prevent or decrease the frequency of outbreaks and reactivation once it's already established.

HSV SUBUNIT VACCINE: HERPEVAC

An HSV-2 subunit vaccine is made using just a portion (subunit) of the HSV particle to trigger an immune response, rather than using the whole virus. These types of vaccines pose no risk of giving herpes infection, because only a part of the virus, usually specially manufactured, is present. GlaxoSmithKline (GSK) is currently pursuing development of such a vaccine, and is now in the midst of a Phase 3 clinical trial of its Herpevac vaccine for women. The National Institutes for Allergy and Infectious Diseases has co-sponsored the study, and the trial has now enrolled more than 7,000 subjects, all of them women between the ages of 18 and 30.

While the Herpevac study is ongoing, results are available from an earlier round of Phase 3 trials of the same GSK HSV-2 subunit vaccine—two double-blind, placebo-controlled studies. Both studies were carried out in *discordant couples,* meaning that one person had genital herpes and one did not. Study participants in the category of *uninfected* tested negative for HSV-2, and the study included some who had not been infected with either HSV-1 or HSV-2.

Interestingly, the GSK study assessed effectiveness in two very different ways. First, the study followed all uninfected subjects closely to see whether they developed any signs or symptoms of disease. Secondly, uninfected partners in the study were tested at intervals to see whether they had *seroconverted,* that is, acquired infection as evidenced by the presence of circulating antibodies to HSV-2.

In the end, the GSK subunit vaccine performed very differently depending on the measure used—and perhaps most important, depending on the segment of the uninfected population studied. Bottom line: The vaccine proved partly successful only in women who had not previously been infected with HSV-1. In this population in the two studies, the risk of developing genital herpes symptoms was reduced by about 75%. The risk of becoming *infected* (seroconversion) was reduced by about 40%. Researchers think this may be because in some persons the immunity stimulated by the vaccine is not sufficient to keep HSV from establishing latent infection but is adequate for reducing the signs and symptoms of HSV if infection occurs.

Why the apparent protective effect only in women—specifically women without prior HSV-1? The question of pre-existing infection and its role has been discussed at length in the research community. Though there are conflicting data on this question, some researchers believe that infection with one viral type usually gives a person partial immunity to the other type, because the two viruses are closely related. By this logic, subjects with prior HSV-1 already carry substantial immunity—immunity the vaccine could not significantly improve upon. The question of why the GSK subunit vaccine proved effective only in *women* also remains a matter of debate. One part of the explanation might be the fact that women are more likely than men to become infected with HSV to begin with. Therefore, in a clinical trial, the female study population will experience a larger number of transmission "events." Logically, then, it is more feasible to demonstrate the statistical significance of an intervention (such as a vaccine) in women than it is in men. It's also possible there are important differences between the sexes in the way the immune system responds to a vaccine.

As of this writing, the current Herpevac clinical trial is expected to produce its initial findings by around 2010. Researchers will be looking closely at outcomes such as prevention of initial HSV infection (seroconversion), prevention of symptomatic genital herpes, and patterns of asymptomatic shedding in those who do become infected. All of these outcomes bear on the public health value of the vaccine.

OTHER VACCINE APPROACHES

The vaccine challenge is daunting. Because the herpes virus stays in the body for the life of the host, scientists are wary of producing vaccines from herpes viruses that are live. Even if the vaccine strain is weakened, there is concern that in some people it could cause disease. In addition, herpes simplex is a large complex virus. The genome encodes about 85 distinct proteins. (By comparison, hepatitis B and HPV have less than 12 proteins; influenza has 8.) It is not known which of these proteins, if any, result in an immune response that protects from infection. And, to make matters more difficult, a number of these HSV genes are designed specifically to fight against immune responses, making HSV a very elusive target.

Nonetheless, there are scores of laboratories across the world involved in experiments that might lead to a herpes vaccine, and some advances are being made. For one, scientists have a growing sophistication in their understanding of the immunology of HSV infection. Traditional immunology emphasizes eliciting neutralizing antibodies against the virus, but other kinds of responses, such as T cell responses, have become better understood. Scientists are now interested in exploring whether and how the cellular immune response causes people to experience herpes in such dramatically different ways. Why is it that one person will have multiple outbreaks and another will never have visible symptoms? If it's the host immune response that is responsible for this variation, can the most successful immune responses be mimicked by a vaccine?

One of the avenues now being explored is the potential advantage of delivering vaccine in a novel way that more directly attacks the virus. HSV replicates in the most superficial layer of the skin, the epidermis. Traditional, intramuscular administration of vaccines may stimulate T cells that migrate to various tissues in the body, but for herpes the goal may be to stimulate T cells that migrate specifically to the skin or to the mucous membranes in the genital tract. One possible strategy for doing this is to give the vaccine intradermally like a TB (tuberculosis) skin test. Animal models suggest this may elicit memory T cells that are better able to home back to the skin. Another potential approach is to give a vaccine orally or intranasally;

these methods may stimulate antibodies that are better able to local-
ize to cervical and vaginal fluid through the concept known as the
common mucosal immune system.

The T cells that fight against HSV are known to move from
blood to skin when a person gets a symptomatic HSV recurrence.
Recently, scientists have been able to stain these HSV-specific T cells
and to see them under the microscope using skin biopsies. One new
finding from these studies is that the T cells called into action to
fight a recurrence actually persist in the local area for several weeks
after HSV lesions heal. Some researchers hypothesize these cells have
local antiviral activity that may eventually decline. Combined with
the new data that HSV asymptomatic reactivation is more frequent
than previously thought when measured with very sensitive tests, the
presence of these post-lesion T cells demonstrates the importance of
the skin as an essential battleground for determining just how symptomatic one's HSV recurrence is likely to be. The search continues
for a topical or systemic therapy that could beef up the immune
response in the most critical layer of the skin system, without leading
to allergies or other problems.

As mentioned earlier, a key hurdle for herpes simplex research
has to do with the nervous system. HSV is able to live in a so-called
latent state in nests of nerve cells termed sensory ganglia. These ganglia lie near, but outside, of the spinal cord and the bony vertebral
column. Previously, the sensory ganglia were thought to be hidden
from the immune system. Recent work, however, has disproved this
assumption. We now know that T cells actively monitor the level of
HSV infection in these sensory ganglia. Researchers in Holland have
removed the sensory ganglia that are involved with typical HSV-1
infection from people who have died. Their findings are that T cells

which can recognize and fight against HSV-1 are specifically localized to these sensory ganglia, and research in an animal model confirms this. This evidence suggests that an effective vaccine has to produce an immune response that will work in more than just the skin.

The vaccine research that has gone the farthest through the cycle of safety and efficacy trials is the Herpevac product described above. While this is a subunit vaccine, researchers are looking at a number of alternate strategies for thwarting HSV, among them:

- **Single Peptide:** HSV encodes 85 long proteins. Peptides are short pieces of these proteins. Utilizing the single peptide approach, would it be effective to take a small synthetic piece of the protein that triggers an immune response and give that as a vaccine? In 2006, researchers published the results of studies that measured immune responses to peptides covering about half of these 85 proteins. As a result, new vaccine candidates incorporating results from these and similar studies are under study in animals.

- **Multiple Peptide:** Perhaps an immune response to a complex virus needs to be complex. What about using a 'string of pearls idea—taking a number of highly antigenic peptides and stringing them together? This idea is actively under investigation.

- **Killed Virus:** What about growing the virus in a control, administering it as a whole, killed virus? It worked against polio, but unfortunately, while attractive, this approach has not worked yet for either therapeutic or preventive vaccine methods against HSV.

• **Attentuated Live Virus:** Several companies are actively investigating this method, which has been successfully used for the varicella zoster (chicken pox/shingles) vaccine. By using genetically mutated live virus, this has the potential to be broadly immunogenic. Although the use of live virus always raises safety concerns, the success against varicella zoster suggests the potential for immunizing against other herpesviruses as well.

Those working in the vaccine development field have many possibilities to explore, but they face complicated trade-offs of safety, complexity, cost, and efficacy. For example, the attenuated live virus approach mentioned above is likely to stimulate a multi-pronged immune response of antibodies and T cells. Concerns remain, however, about the safety of injecting persons with a weakened virus that may still be capable of setting up a latent infection. Meanwhile, subunit vaccines like Herpevac are stable and well defined, but are difficult to administer in a fashion that stimulates a strong T cell response. The 'slam dunk' has so far proved elusive.

Researchers say the field is also hampered by the lack of an animal model that has human-like recurrence patterns, and by unanswered questions about individual variations in host immunity. They still don't know what it is about the immune system of people with low HSV shedding that sets them apart from people with frequent lesions and symptoms.

On the positive side, however, vaccine development has been invigorated by the success of the HPV vaccines developed by Merck and GlaxoSmithKline. These use synthetic "virus-like particles" rather than live virus but have achieved near 100% efficacy against an infection which is similar to HSV in its predilection for the epidermis or superficial genital epithelium. In addition, as of this writing there are important studies in Africa evaluating the role of HSV-2 in the spread of HIV. Most notably, researchers are testing the concept of making people less susceptible to HIV by suppressing genital herpes with acyclovir. The basis for this approach is the high prevalence of HSV-2 in areas with HIV epidemics and research that shows HSV-2 facilitates the spread of HIV. If acyclovir can have a demonstrated impact, the drive for an HSV-2 vaccine might gain important new support—and funding—around the globe.

NOVEL THERAPEUTIC AGENTS

But what, you may ask, about a *real cure*? What about something that doesn't just slow down HSV but kills it? Where is the medical innovation that would help people who already have herpes—not just the uninfected?

There are, in fact, a large number of researchers investigating completely new approaches to HSV, including chemical compounds that may one day prove useful in new medications. In 2002 there were two well-publicized scientific articles that heralded new compounds called *helicase-primase inhibitors* that could speed the healing of HSV lesions in animal studies and reduce the severity and frequency of recurrences. These compounds are entering early human trials that will determine how safe they are and whether they work to treat HSV infections.

The thing to keep in mind if you see a news clip suggesting a revolutionary breakthrough is that the process of bringing a new drug to market is long, expensive, and complex. Test-tube experiments are followed by laboratory tests on animals, which are then followed by exhaustive tests or "clinical trials" in humans. These trials—organized in three separate phases—focus first on safety, and later on both the safety and effectiveness of the drug in question.

According to the U.S. Pharmaceutical Manufacturers Association, only 1 in 5,000 new chemicals investigated by the industry ever makes it to the drugstore. It also estimates that the average new drug takes 10–15 years to bring to market. An independent study by Tufts Center for the Study of Drug Development says the cost of the development process averages roughly $900 million per drug. The path is full of pitfalls, and there are a myriad of would-be miracle drugs left by the wayside every year.

While herpes is not public health priority number one these days, it's worth mentioning that a major herpes breakthrough of any kind is potentially worth a lot of money. For example, with millions of symptomatic herpes patients in the United States alone, any treatment or diagnostic test has the potential for major commercial success. Today's herpes drugs already have proved to be blockbusters, with Valtrex® yielding sales of over $1 billion in 2006. This is both an incentive and disincentive to potential developers. Clearly the market is substantial, and a breakthrough drug would stand to make money. On the other hand, with safe and effective antivirals already established—and with all of them likely to be available as generics by 2010—the product would have to pose a major gain over the current drugs in order to be a cost-effective investment.

The point is that herpes is not a lost and forgotten infection in the realm of biomedical research. If you have herpes, and you're anxious to hear about important scientific advances, there are any number of medical journals and texts that report on new developments. Many of these are summarized for lay audiences in *The Helper,* a quarterly newsletter of the American Social Health Association. (See the Resource List on page 221 for details.)

WHAT YOU CAN DO

It is important to recognize that all advances in the development of treatments or vaccines for genital herpes are achieved only if people are willing to volunteer for clinical research. Any new research is initially done in the test tube, then in animals, and only if a compound appears safe can it progress to trials in people. Those who volunteer for studies that test new drugs do it for several reasons. One is they hope to receive treatment that is effective for their condition, or an intervention that will protect them from infection, as in the case of vaccine research. But they also want to make a contribution to science and to society—a form of altruism that's essential for all medical progress. Some people feel that this is a way to give back to society for effective medical care they have received, or in hope that more effective care may be developed for future generations. If you are interested in participating in clinical research, you may want to look at http://www.clinicaltrials.gov, a Web site maintained by National Institutes of Health which lists clinical trials by conditions (you can type "herpes" in the search box); or, if you live near a medical school, look at its Web site.

18

OTHER SEXUALLY TRANSMITTED INFECTIONS

Although herpes is the principal subject of our book, it's just one component of a broader epidemic of sexually transmitted infections (STIs) in this country. The Centers for Disease Control and Prevention (CDC) estimates there were more than 19 million new STI cases (including herpes) in the U.S. in 2005—almost half of them among young people between the ages of 15 and 24. Perhaps another way to appreciate the frequency of these infections is to consider the fact that more than 50% of Americans will have at least one STI in their lifetime. Direct medical costs associated with STIs are estimated by CDC at up to $14.1 billion annually. While some of these are bacterial infections and easily cured, others are viral infections for which no cure presently exists. Several are on the rise. When you're discussing issues of sexual health with a current or prospective sex partner, both of you should be considering the broader spectrum of sexually transmitted infections. Women *especially* need to protect themselves because of the associated increased risks of an impaired ability to have children and injury to the newborn.

A note on terminology: When we discuss the presence of infection in a specific community or in the general population, we use the terms *prevalence* and *incidence.* Prevalence is how many people in the population have a given disease at any given time. Incidence is the number of new cases occurring in a certain time period. For example, we believe approximately 50 million people in the U.S. are currently infected with herpes; that's our number for prevalence. We expect at least 1 million new cases to be added to that number each year, so 1 million is the annual incidence. In the summaries of other STIs that follow, we will be talking about annual incidence (the number of new cases per year) unless otherwise noted.

CHLAMYDIA — A bacterium, *Chlamydia trachomatis,* is transmitted to an estimated 3 million people in the U.S. each year. Antibiotics can rid the body of chlamydia in a matter of days, but people with chlamydia often fail to get prompt treatment because they have no idea they're infected. The reason is that chlamydia causes no signs or symptoms of illness in up to 50% of men and 75% of women. When symptoms are present, they often include painful urination for men and vaginal discharge for women. Unfortunately, the scarcity of obvious symptoms doesn't mean chlamydia is harmless. Left untreated, it can cause a variety of reproductive problems. In women, it can lead to pelvic inflammatory disease (PID), which can cause fallopian tube or uterine damage. This in turn can lead to infertility and ectopic pregnancy. Chlamydia is so common that if you're a sexually active woman, with multiple partners, the CDC strongly recommends you have a *screening test at least once a year.* All sexually active women under the age of 26 should also be tested annually. Severe complications in men are uncommon but do occur.

GONORRHEA — You might think of gonorrhea as a sort of dinosaur STI, one that was a problem decades ago but has since been brought under control. Not so. The annual incidence (the number of new cases per year) declined steadily from 1975 through 1997, according to CDC, but recent years have seen a resurgence. Total new cases are estimated at more than 700,000 per year. The rate of infection is especially high among teenagers and minorities. The symptoms are similar to those of chlamydia, and people who are infected, especially women, can be completely without symptoms. Most cases are easily cured with antibiotics. But as with chlamydia, left untreated, gonorrhea can lead to reproductive tract infections associated with pelvic inflammatory disease, ectopic pregnancy, and infertility. Men also can suffer reproductive damage.

SYPHILIS— Public health officials have been making a concerted effort to eliminate syphilis in the U.S. and have had much success. The CDC estimates there were fewer than 6,000 cases of primary or secondary syphilis in the year 2000—down 30% from 1997 figures. Subsequent years, however, saw syphilis outbreaks in various populations, and the national rates are again rising. From 2004 to 2005, the syphilis rate actually increased by 11%, bringing the number of primary syphilis cases to 8,724. Running a complicated course once inside the human body, syphilis first causes noticeable ulcers on the genitals, which in some cases may resemble herpes lesions. Untreated, syphilis will seem to disappear spontaneously, but the disease actually goes into a latent phase that can be followed by increasingly serious health complications and death. The complications include problems with the central nervous system or with the heart and blood vessels. The good news: Once diagnosed, syphilis is usually easily cured with antibiotics.

HUMAN PAPILLOMAVIRUS (HPV) — You have probably heard a good deal about HPV in the last few years. It is one of the most common sexually transmitted infections, and in 2006 the FDA approved an HPV vaccine. Based on 2003-2004 data, prevalence nationwide was estimated at 26.8% among females between the ages of 14 and 59, with the highest prevalence in the 20-24 year-old age group.

There are more than 100 types of HPV, about three dozen of which can affect the genital area. Among the many types of genital HPV, some may cause minor cell changes such as warts. These are called "low-risk types." If warts are present, they can be treated in a number of ways. Other types of HPV can cause the kinds of cell changes on the cervix that are usually detected by Pap tests. These are called "high-risk types" because they increase the risk of cervical cancer. But it is important to remember that the overwhelming majority of women who have high-risk types *do not* develop cervical cancer— or even have abnormal Pap results.

HPV can defy treatment and persist for years, though there's also evidence that the immune system sometimes clears the virus over time. There are several different treatments that remove genital warts or remove the affected tissue on the cervix, but treatment isn't certain to eradicate the virus. Genital warts, in particular, often recur after treatment.

Diagnostic tests can be run on Pap test specimens or other cervical samples to determine if genital HPV types are present. These tests are being used with increasing frequency, and in women 30 and older they are recommended as an adjunct test with all Pap tests.

The other good news is that the Merck HPV vaccine licensed in 2006 can prevent initial infection with the two types of HPV (6, 11) most likely to cause visible warts and the types most likely to cause cervical cancer (16, 18). While the vaccine is primarily targeted to females 11 and 12 years of age, catch-up vaccination is recommended for women 13-26. A second manufacturer, GlaxoSmithKline, is also expected to have approval for its HPV vaccine in 2007.

HEPATITIS B — Hepatitis B virus (HBV) is a form of hepatitis (liver infection) which is most commonly transmitted by sex. HBV infections are spread through body fluids such as blood, semen, or vaginal fluids. The CDC estimates about 51,000 new cases per year, of which roughly 55% are sexually transmitted. Other major routes of transmission include the sharing of needles by injecting drug users and accidental needle-sticks among healthcare workers. People who contract HBV can develop chronic liver disease entailing liver cell damage, cirrhosis, and increased risk for liver cancer. HBV infection cannot be cured, and there are an estimated 1.25 million people currently living with chronic hepatitis B infection. Vaccines to prevent HBV infection have been licensed since 1981, and CDC recommends vaccination for all infants, children, adolescents and sexually active adults.

HIV/AIDS — You probably already know more about HIV infection and AIDS than we can possibly cover here, but it's nevertheless important to include. HIV is, after all, transmitted primarily through unprotected sexual intercourse, so the precautions required for other STIs can also help to prevent the spread of HIV. As with so many other viral infections, symptoms may not show up until years after the virus takes hold. The symptoms are extremely diverse, mimicking dozens of other illnesses. HIV attacks the immune system itself, wrecking the body's natural defenses against a host of different infections. There are treatments to slow this assault against the immune system, but as yet none suppresses it completely. The total number of new HIV infections in the United States is estimated at 800,000-900,000, with approximately 40,000 new infections each year.

While the infections listed above are the most troublesome STIs in many ways, others are worth mentioning as well. Common parasites such as *Trichomonas vaginalis,* a frequent cause of vaginitis (inflammation of the vaginal tissue), are often transmitted sexually—to the tune of 7.4 million new infections annually. There are a dozen other infections easily spread through intimate contact, including sex. These include scabies and pubic lice. Bacterial vaginosis (BV), the most common vaginal infection in the United States, affects about 16 percent of women. Not strictly an STI, BV is an imbalance between the types of bacteria normally found in a woman's vagina. It has a number of causes, and is sometimes associated with having new or multiple sex partners.

If you want more information about any or all sexually transmitted infections, there are a number of resources at hand. Although not all Web sites have up-to-date information, several first-rate sites are profiled in the Resource List at the end of this book. One major source of help is free of charge and as convenient as the nearest telephone: The STI Resource Center. (See Resource List, page 221, for this and other useful phone numbers and Web sites.) There is also a free information service through the CDC, which offers confidential information and referrals, including print materials sent free of charge to your home address. It also can tell you the location of a STI clinic run by the public health department in your community. Testing and treatment for STIs is often free or inexpensive.

AN OUNCE OF PREVENTION

STIs are transmitted in a variety of ways, but a few principles of prevention apply equally to almost all of them:

• Vaccination is the first line of defense against infectious diseases. Tens of millions of sexually active adults still have not been vaccinated against hepatitis B. And young women now have the option of vaccination against four genital HPV types.

• Most STIs can have mild or unrecognized symptoms. Therefore you can't assume that a lack of symptoms equals a clean bill of health.

• Testing for the leading STIs is not a routine part of regular healthcare for most people. Don't assume you have been tested for everything. Ask your healthcare provider about specific tests for chlamydia, gonorrhea, HIV, and herpes. In addition, for women, a combination of regular Pap tests and HPV testing when needed will help to protect against any possible complications of HPV infection.

• If you're free of infection yourself, your risk is zero if you have sex only with one *uninfected* partner, who in turn has sex only with you. As soon as either partner has a new sexual contact, however, all bets are off. With so many STIs that show no symptoms, how do you know who is infected and who isn't?

• What if you don't really know your partner well and certainly don't know about his or her past? Those having sex with a partner who *might* be carrying an STI, or with several such partners, can dramatically reduce their risk of getting or spreading an STI by using latex or plastic condoms for each and every act of sexual intercourse—whether the penetration is oral, vaginal, or anal. Condoms used in this way are very effective prevention for chlamydia, gonorrhea, syphilis, hepatitis, and HIV. The risk of HPV and herpes is also decreased in people who consistently and correctly use condoms. Condoms can lower the risk of herpes by about 50%, for both men and women.

HERPES AND OTHER STIS

Some people with herpes question whether they are at greater risk of getting other illnesses because of HSV. Some assume that a person with one virus in the herpes family will be prone to get all of them. Others have seen press coverage that implies herpes might somehow mutate into the AIDS virus or that herpes itself will damage the immune system or cause cancer.

On all of these points, the facts should be reassuring. Because all the herpesviruses are quite common, you may host herpes simplex and several other members of the family as well, such as Epstein-Barr and varicella zoster. But having HSV in no way dooms you to getting all the herpesviruses; each one is transmitted separately. Nor does having HSV mean that you have a deficient immune system.

Lastly, herpes does not cause cancer, nor does it turn into HIV, although it may make a person more susceptible to contracting HIV. Actually, several of the other STIs mentioned in this chapter are also considered risk factors for HIV. Chlamydia, gonorrhea, syphilis—the presence of any of these infections increases the risk of acquiring HIV, *if and when* there is sexual contact with an HIV-infected person. But none of them by itself leads to HIV. (By the way, it's probable that a person with HIV is more infectious if he or she has another STI as well.)

WHAT YOU CAN DO

If you have herpes, you now know that sexually transmitted infections are a factor in your life as well as in millions of other lives. If you feel you need more information about STIs, you can call the CDC. See Resources, page 221, for more information about STIs, for free written materials, or a referral to a health-care provider in your community. If you feel you may have been exposed to other STIs through unprotected sex, or if you have symptoms that resemble those of a common STI, talk to your healthcare provider about it. There are tests for all the infections listed here. And as always, early treatment is the key to avoiding serious medical complications.

MANAGING HERPES

19

LEGAL ISSUES

"I was dating this girl, and we slept together once," says a caller to the National Herpes Hotline. "Now I've got herpes, and I'm thinking about taking legal action. I'm sure I got it from her. Is there any way I can prove it?"

If you've already read the first 18 chapters of this book, you know that this caller has a lot to learn about herpes, starting with the fact that he probably can't be sure how he became infected at all. This uncertainty is pretty common with regard to other STIs as well.

Lawsuits waged by one person against another over sexually transmitted infections are often pointless. Not only is it difficult (if not impossible) to prove when and from whom the injured party contracted a particular STI, it may be equally difficult to establish that the "guilty" party even knew he or she was infected. What's more, such cases invade the privacy of both plaintiff and defendant and can be wrenching experiences for everyone involved. Nonetheless, while it is often difficult to prove the source of infection, there are criminal and civil laws designed to prevent a person from knowingly exposing another person to an STI such as herpes without that person's knowledge or consent. And because lawsuits involving the transmission of genital herpes are brought to court with some regularity, readers of this book may find it helpful to learn a bit about the legal landscape.

CRIMINAL LAW AND INFECTIOUS DISEASES

Knowingly exposing a person to a sexually transmitted infection such as genital herpes can be considered a *criminal offense* in some jurisdictions. Criminal law is found in statutes that have been enacted by state legislatures or by the U.S. Congress. These laws are enforced by the government (police and prosecutors) and violations can be punished with imprisonment or fines.

A number of states have passed laws making it a crime to knowingly pass HIV (the AIDS virus) to another person. In fact, the original Ryan White Act of 1990, which provides emergency AIDS grants to states, required states receiving those funds to make it a crime for HIV-infected people not to tell potential sex partners about their HIV status.

There are also criminal laws that apply to sexually transmitted infections other than HIV/AIDS. About one quarter of the states have laws criminalizing the transmission of genital herpes. Some of these laws apply to any "communicable disease" or "venereal disease" (terms that would be interpreted to include genital herpes), while others specifically mention genital herpes. All of these laws make *knowingly* transmitting herpes a *misdemeanor,* which is less serious than a *felony* and punishable with fines or jail sentences of less than one year. Following physician-recommended practices for preventing transmission might be a defense for a person charged under one of these laws.

CIVIL LAWS AND INFECTIOUS DISEASES

Beyond the possibility of criminal penalties, a person who knowingly transmits an infection such as genital herpes may be sued under common law tort principles. A "tort" is, literally, a "wrong." Tort laws, like many other *civil (non-criminal)* laws are generally not embodied in statutes but instead are shaped by judges. In contrast to criminal law, the plaintiff in such cases is usually an individual, and money is often the major issue. Thus, if Jimmy wrongs Johnny, Johnny can sue in tort, and it's up to the court to decide if Johnny is entitled to monetary compensation.

How do the courts make such determinations? Courts draw on legal, moral, economic, and public policy principles that have been developed and applied by courts in previous cases. Tort law is largely left up to the individual states, and the rules can vary quite a bit from one state to another.

People have long been held liable in civil cases for exposing others to infectious diseases such as tuberculosis and whooping cough. In 1896, for example, the Wisconsin Supreme Court ruled that an employer should have told a servant that the employer's child was sick with typhoid fever before making the servant clean the child's room. And in a 1920 case, *Crowell v. Crowell,* the North Carolina Supreme Court held that a man was liable for fraudulently concealing from his bride that he had syphilis.

In the modern era, the same type of legal argument has been applied to infectious agents such as HIV, herpes simplex, and human papillomavirus (HPV). Lawsuits over sexually transmitted infections have been on the rise since the mid-1980s. Because of its deadly consequences, lawsuits involving HIV infection have attracted greater publicity than other STI cases, but there have been some heavily publicized herpes cases as well. Given the complex patchwork of state and local jurisdictions, no one knows how many STI lawsuits are pending at any given time, but experts say that only a small percentage ever reach the courtroom.

THE LEGAL FRAMEWORK

If and when someone decides to take legal action after becoming infected with an STI, he or she can make use of the criminal or civil laws that prohibit the knowing transmissions of such infections. Filing a criminal complaint will permit the police to investigate the facts alleged to see whether a crime has been committed. Instead of, or in addition to, filing a criminal complaint, an individual infected with herpes may choose to file a tort lawsuit against the person who transmitted the infection.

Lawsuits over STIs may be based on one or more legal claims, including *assault, battery, infliction of emotional distress, fraud, misrepresentation,* or *negligence.* Regardless of the specific theoretical basis, however, most of these cases hinge on the same factual questions: Did the defendant know he or she had an STI? If not, did he or she take reasonable care to discover this condition? Did he or she withhold this information? And in doing so, did the defendant either accidentally or intentionally harm an innocent person?

While courts in various states might differ on the subtleties of interpretation in STI cases, a growing number of cases decided in the last two decades have reached the same two conclusions: 1) a person has a legal right to know about the health of a sex partner, and 2) a person with an infection like genital herpes has a legal duty to prevent its spread. In *R.A.P. v. B.J.P.,* for example, the Minnesota Supreme Court recognized the right of a man to sue his ex-wife for negligence and fraud because she slept with him without informing him she had genital herpes. Thus, in the eyes of one court, those with an STI have, at a minimum, a duty to disclose that fact to those with whom they are sexually intimate. Lying to conceal an STI is often considered a form of *intentional infliction of harm*. Simply failing to tell a partner about an STI, on the other hand, is more likely to be viewed as an act of *negligence*.

By the very nature of the supposed wrongdoing, cases involving the transmission of STIs are difficult to prove. Things were said or not said, precautions were taken or not taken—all in the heat of passion and rarely before witnesses.

In terms of physical evidence, the plaintiff often has a tough time establishing causation—proving that the defendant was the cause of the plaintiff's infection. With herpes, as we know, the infection may be acquired months or years before symptoms appear or are recognized. And more than half of all transmission occurs when a partner is asymptomatic or has symptoms but doesn't recognize them as herpes. If the plaintiff has had more than one partner, it may be impossible to prove that an infection came from a particular person. Pinpointing the source is, at the very least, difficult, and medical evidence must be supported by laboratory documentation of a first episode of HSV infection.

COMMON DEFENSES AND STRATEGIES

Tracing the source of other sexually transmitted infections can be equally challenging, so most defendants in STI cases avail themselves of expert opinion to challenge the proof of the claims made against them. As part of this process, the sexual past of the plaintiff often becomes an issue. The defense attorney will probably ask detailed questions about the plaintiff's prior sexual history and may well overstep our usual notions of privacy and propriety.

In addition, defense lawyers in some of these cases have used strategies to question the very basis of the lawsuit. There have been cases, for example, in which a defendant was able to avoid liability for transmitting an STI because it was a criminal offense in certain states for people to have sexual relations outside of marriage (defined legally as *fornication*), and courts have sometimes ruled that a plaintiff cannot recover damages for any harm or injury that resulted from an illegal act. As interpreted by the U.S. Supreme Court in its 2003 decision *Lawrence v. Texas,* however, fornication laws violate the federal constitutional right of privacy. In that decision, the Court held that adults have the right to make decisions about private, consensual, intimate relationships without intrusion from the government. The Virginia Supreme Court struck down that state's fornication law in *Martin v. Ziherl,* a 2005 case involving a lawsuit over the transmission of herpes. The plaintiff was then able to pursue the original tort lawsuit against the defendant who allegedly gave her herpes. While a small number of states still have laws on the books that criminalize fornication, these would also be declared unconstitutional if challenged.

Another defense sometimes raised in herpes transmission cases is interspousal immunity, a doctrine that says spouses cannot sue one another. This doctrine is recognized in some jurisdictions but not in others; where it is recognized, a husband or wife who contracts herpes from a spouse has no recourse in civil law.

Other defenses like "marital privilege" or the right of privacy have been generally unsuccessful. In general, the courts have ruled that unmarried persons can sue their sexual partners. In a leading case involving transmission of genital herpes, *Kathleen K. v. Robert B.,* the defendant argued that single people do not have a relationship of trust and confidence like married people and thus have no right to full disclosure of an infection. The court, however, ruled that intimate acts imply such a relationship. The court also rejected the defendant's argument that the plaintiff had assumed the risk of getting an STI by consenting to intercourse; in the court's view, consent to intercourse is *not* consent to being infected with an STI.

This last point is perhaps the most hotly contested in the legal arena. Some defense attorneys have been able to argue persuasively that anyone who has unprotected sexual intercourse in today's society, or who fails to ask about the sexual health of a partner, is equally responsible for infections that may be transmitted sexually, especially during a one night stand. In less casual relationships, however, the courts are more likely to see a lack of candor as an actionable breach of trust.

Lawyers have found a great many subtleties in STI cases, and the legal landscape is still taking shape. The availability of drugs to reduce outbreaks and thus the risk of transmission may still affect the legal standards governing transmission. Regardless of how the law evolves, however, there is a clear consensus about the legal importance of honest disclosure. If someone with an STI tells his or her partner about the infection and gives the partner a choice about sexual involvement, grounds for legal action are vastly reduced. If, on the other hand, someone lies about or conceals the truth about an infection, there is ample precedent to suggest he or she might be vulnerable to civil or criminal penalties.

HERPES AND HEALTH INSURANCE

People diagnosed with herpes sometimes raise questions about health insurance and the potential for discrimination against those infected with herpes. Overall, the news here is good. For the nearly two-thirds of Americans covered under a group plan as part of their employee benefits, herpes generally is no issue at all. Millions of people with genital HSV routinely submit claims for office visits, prescription medication, and sometimes counseling. There may be limits placed on coverage under any particular policy, but herpes is seldom, if ever, regarded as different from other medical conditions.

For individuals who get health insurance through an employer's group plan, the chance of being discriminated against on the basis of a herpes infection is very small. The Health Insurance Portability and Accountability Act of 1996 (HIPAA) prohibits group health plans from excluding coverage for individuals based on their health status. HIPAA also does not permit plans to exclude coverage for pre-existing conditions for more than 12 months and requires that they credit previously carried insurance against that waiting period.

Problems do sometimes emerge, however, for people who seek health insurance for themselves outside employer-based group plans. If you're applying for coverage as part of an individual or family plan, you may have to file a detailed application that includes questions about STIs. And for some insurers, a history of herpes or other sexually transmitted infections may prompt further questions.

Some plans will regard herpes as a *pre-existing condition,* just as they would many other illnesses. In this case, they would enroll you but would exclude herpes-related claims until some waiting period has passed. Others may accept you as a plan member but attach a *rider* to the policy that excludes coverage for herpes altogether. There's also a small chance that your application may be rejected.

Currently, most insurance companies examine individual applications on a case-by-case basis and make decisions according to a variety of factors. Industry sources say that a history of herpes alone would seldom be grounds for denying coverage. It's also important to remember that herpes claims have almost insignificant cost when compared with diabetes, heart disease, and many other ailments.

Once a person has insurance, there are laws in most states prohibiting insurance carriers from refusing to renew or canceling their policies unless the claimant fails to pay, commits fraud or misrepresentation, fails to comply with provisions of the plan, leaves the service area, or leaves the organization offering the plan. These laws should prevent an insurer from canceling coverage for a person simply because he or she has acquired and sought treatment for herpes.

Anyone who has questions about health insurance or about discrimination in this area can take one of several steps:

• Work with an experienced, independent insurance agent who knows the insurance companies in your state and can provide a list of companies with good credentials.

• Consumers can contact the A. M. Best Company for annually updated ratings of life and health insurers. (Ratings reflect the financial stability of these companies.) A. M. Best can be reached at (908) 439-2200 or at www.ambest.com.

• Some states have *open enrollment programs* in which applicants cannot be denied coverage for medical reasons. Your state insurance commission or department of insurance will have detailed information about these.

• If you have problems getting coverage, you can appeal the insurance company's decision in writing. You also have the legal right of access to your MIB (Medical Information Bureau) file, which insurers routinely review as part of their background check on individuals applying for coverage. MIB, Inc., is a nonprofit industry "alliance" whose membership comprises more than 600 health insurance companies. It was originally established to root out fraudulent health insurance claims. MIB keeps files on only a small percentage of insured individuals. To find out if you have an MIB file and to obtain a copy if you do, you will need to call 866-692-6901 (or 866-346-3642 for the hearing-impaired). MIB offers this service free of charge once annually. We recommend that you learn more about how this request is filed, and also find detailed information on the organization, by visiting the MIB Web site, at www.mib.com. Their mailing address is MIB, Inc., P. O. Box 105, Essex Station, Boston, MA 02112.

RESOURCE LIST

ASHA SERVICES AND MATERIALS
American Social Health Association (ASHA)
P. O. Box 13827
Research Triangle Park, NC 27709-3827

Since 1914, the American Social Health Association (ASHA) has been dedicated to improving the health of individuals, families, and communities, with a focus on preventing sexually transmitted infections (STIs) and their harmful consequences. ASHA has pursued its mission through education, communication, advocacy and policy analysis activities. These are designed to heighten public, patient, provider, policymaker and media awareness of STI prevention, screening, diagnosis and treatment strategies.

ASHA publishes materials to provide a valuable resource for accurate medical information and emotional support for those affected by sexually transmitted infections.

NATIONAL HERPES HOTLINE: 919-361-8488
Established in 1979, the National Herpes Hotline operates Monday through Friday, 9 am to 8 pm, Eastern Time. Information specialists are available to address questions related to diagnosis, transmission, prevention, and treatment of herpes simplex virus.

STI Resource Hotline: 1-800-227-8922

The STI Resource Center Hotline is a program of the American Social Health Association (ASHA) that provides information, materials and referrals to anyone concerned about sexually transmitted infections (STI). Health Communication Specialists are on staff to answer STI questions on such topics as transmission, risk reduction, prevention, testing and treatment. The service receives more than 180,000 calls a year and is not supported by state or federal funds, but by donations from foundations, corporations and individuals such as yourself.

This Hotline is open from 9:00 am to 8:00 pm, Eastern Time, Monday through Friday.

Combined with the high public demand, it is sometimes difficult to get through to speak to a Health Communication Specialist. Please feel free to look through our online STI information section at: http://www.ashastd.org/learn/learn_overview.cfm to find answers to questions you may have.

STI Message Board

ASHA now offers an interactive STI Message Board that allows users to ask questions and interact with others in a confidential, supportive environment. The board, which is moderated by ASHA staff, includes a specific forum dedicated to herpes discussions.

www.ashastd.org/phpbb/index.php

ASHA Web Sites
STI Information: Herpes Resource Center - www.ASHAstd.org
For Teens: www.iwannaknow.org
Español: www.quierosaber.org

ASHA Online Product Catalog
ASHA has an online catalog with products for individuals and healthcare providers, such as patient education brochures, books and posters. All products are available for secure online ordering at:
www.ashastd.org/commerce/webstore/index.cfm

If you are a healthcare provider and wish to receive a free print catalog of patient education materials, please call, ASHA Catalog Customer Service at 1-800-783-9877

INFORMATION ON MEDICATIONS

United States Food and Drug Administration (FDA) Office of Consumer Affairs
Rockville, MD
1 888 463-6332
www.fda.gov
The FDA provides information on a wide array of topics, including prescription medications, over-the-counter drugs, dietary supplements, vaccines, and medical devices (including condoms). Of particular note is the Drug Information Hotline of the FDA Center for Drug Evaluation and Research (301) 827-4573.

GlaxoSmithKline (GSK)

www.herpeshelp.com

As the maker of the antiviral medication Valtrex®, GlaxoSmith-kline maintains a Web site with helpful information.

Novartis Pharmaceuticals

(866) 326-8471

www.famvir.com

Consumer information about the antiviral medication Famvir® is available from Novartis Pharmaceuticals through the Web sites and hotline listed above.

OTHER RESOURCES

For diagnostic tests:

STDWEB.COM

Sells confidential STD diagnostics test kits directly to individuals.

University of Washington

(206) 598-6066 (healthcare providers only)

http://depts.washington.edu/herpes/

For support and counseling:

American Association of Marriage and Family Therapists

Washington, DC

(202) 452-0109, 9 am – 5 pm, ET, M - F

www.aamft.org

The Association provides information through the mail about

therapists in your area. Referrals are for solution-oriented therapy/counseling.

For reproductive health/family planning questions:
PLANNED PARENTHOOD FEDERATION OF AMERICA
www.plannedparenthood.org

For information about insurance companies:
A. M. BEST CO.
(908) 439-2200
www.ambest.com
This organization provides financial stability ratings of approximately 1,500 insurers.

For information about alternative treatments:
THE NATIONAL CENTER FOR COMPLEMENTARY AND ALTERNATIVE MEDICINE (NCCAM)
http://nccam.nih.gov

NATIONAL INSTITUTES OF HEALTH (NIH)
(888) 644-6226
http://nccam.nih.gov
NCCAM explores complementary and alternative healing practices in the context of rigorous science and disseminates authoritative information. Its clearinghouse produces fact sheets, a newsletter and other publications that provide information about research supported by the NCCAM and other centers of the NIH. Information is free of charge and can be ordered through the toll-free number above.

HERPES-RELATED WEB SITES

There are dozens of Web sites offering resources for people with genital herpes, but Web surfers cannot always count on the quality of the information presented. The sites listed here are among the most thorough, with an emphasis on content grounded in published scientific research.

AMERICAN SOCIAL HEALTH ASSOCIATION (ASHA)
www.ashastd.org/herpes/herpes_overview.cfm

ASHA's online Herpes Resource Center offers an in-depth FAQ section, STI Message Board, an e-mail service to answer specific questions, and access to online ordering for print materials on herpes. For a much more complete listing of sites, check the Links page on the ASHA Web site.

AMERICAN HERPES FOUNDATION
www.herpes-foundation.org

Information and resources for patients and medical professionals.

HERPESWEB
www.herpesweb.net

Well-designed international site with patient resources, personal accounts.

INTERNATIONAL HERPES ALLIANCE
www.herpesalliance.com

Educational pages, news, resources, and personal accounts from patients around the world.

International Herpes Management Forum
www.ihmf.org

International academic organization that addresses the clinical care of all major herpesvirus infections. Includes HSV information for patient and professional.

National Institutes of Health (NIH)
www.niaid.nih.gov/factsheets/stdherp.htm

or www.nih.gov

The consumer–oriented "Healthfinder" service available through the NIH Web site offers a question-and-answer page geared to those diagnosed with genital herpes.

U. S. Centers for Disease Control and Prevention (CDC)
http://www.cdc.gov/std/Herpes/default.htm

CDC's Sexually Transmitted Diseases Branch publishes a herpes fact sheet online, along with a bibliography of references and a listing of resources.

WebMD Herpes Information
http://my.webmd.com

WebMD Herpes Message Board
http://boards.webmd.com

Message board discussion on herpes, sex and relationships, with questions answered by herpes expert Terri Warren, R.N., A.N.P., M.S.

GLOSSARY

ACUTE OR EPISODIC THERAPY: Use of medication to relieve symptoms or hasten healing for an individual herpes outbreak.

ANTIBODIES: Elements of the body's immune response, antibodies circulate in the blood and in other bodily fluids to fight disease-causing microbes.

ANTIGEN: Any foreign substance in the body, such as a fragment of a virus, that triggers the immune system to respond with antibodies or other parts of the immune defense system.

ASYMPTOMATIC REACTIVATION, ASYMPTOMATIC SHEDDING: An event in which latent herpes simplex virus reactivates at the nerve root and travels to a skin surface or mucous membrane, yet causes neither signs nor symptoms of infection that can be readily identified by the patient or a medical professional.

ASYMPTOMATIC TRANSMISSION: The spread of virus from one person to another during a period of asymptomatic shedding.

AUTOINOCULATION: The spread of HSV from one part of the body to another. This can result when a person with active herpes deposits a significant amount of virus onto some other vulnerable part of the body—most often a mucous membrane.

CELL CULTURE (VIRAL CULTURE): A diagnostic test for many kinds of viruses. In a cell culture for HSV, a swab of the patient's herpes lesion is placed in a laboratory dish containing normal skin cells to see if HSV will grow.

CELLULAR IMMUNE RESPONSE: The portion of the body's immune response that involves T-lymphocytes—specialized or other cells designed to fight an "antigen" or invading microbe.

DISSEMINATED INFECTION: A herpes infection that spreads over a wider than usual area of the body, frequently afflicting internal organs.

FIRST EPISODE: The body's first encounter with a particular type of herpes simplex, an event that often produces marked symptoms. There are two types of "first episodes." A primary first episode describes the symptoms that appear in the person who has never been infected with either HSV-1 or HSV-2 before. It's sometimes called a "true primary," and it tends to be most severe.

"Nonprimary first episode" describes the symptoms that occur in the person who has been infected first with one type of HSV and then later infected with the second. For example, a person who is infected with HSV-1 and then years later infected with HSV-2 can be said to have a "first episode" of HSV-2 if he or she has symptoms.

"First recognized recurrence" describes the first episode of genital herpes in a person who has had the infection for some time but has not noticed the symptoms in the past.

GANGLION: A knot-like grouping of the nerves that serve a particular part of the body.

GENITAL HERPES: "Genital herpes" can cause symptoms in a variety of sites below the waist. This term is used to denote all HSV infection that is latent in the sacral ganglion, at the base of the spine.

HSV: Abbreviation for herpes simplex virus. HSV-1 denotes herpes simplex type 1, the usual cause of herpes around the mouth or face ("cold sores," "fever blisters"); HSV-2 denotes herpes simplex type 2, the usual cause of recurrent genital herpes.

HERPES ENCEPHALITIS: A rare severe illness that occurs when the brain becomes infected with HSV.

HERPES GLADIATORUM: The presence of herpes lesions on the body skin caused by HSV infection that is transmitted usually through the abrasion of skin in a contact sport, such as wrestling.

HERPETIC WHITLOW: The presence of herpes lesions on the fingers or toes near the nailbed.

HERPESVIRUS: Any one of eight known members of the human herpesvirus family: herpes simplex type 1; herpes simplex type 2; varicella zoster virus; Epstein-Barr virus; cytomegalovirus; human herpes virus type 6; human herpes virus type 7; and human herpes virus type 8.

LATENCY: The phenomenon by which HSV can persist in the nerve roots in an inactive state but retain the capacity to reactivate intermittently and cause viral shedding and lesions.

LESION: A very general term denoting any abnormality on the surface of the body, whether on the skin or on a mucous membrane. Includes sores, pimples, tumors, and more.

MENINGITIS: An inflammation of the meninges, the protective covering around the brain, usually accompanied by stiff neck and extra sensitivity to light. Septic meningitis, caused by bacteria, can be a serious condition and must be treated immediately. Aseptic meningitis, associated with viral infections such as HSV and other causes, generally resolves by itself.

OCULAR HERPES: Symptoms caused by herpes infection in the eyes.

ORAL-FACIAL HERPES: The presence of latent herpes simplex infection in the trigeminal ganglion, at the top of the spine. When reactivated, oral-facial herpes can cause symptoms anywhere on mouth or face—typically cold sores on the lips. Recurrent oral-facial herpes is caused almost exclusively by HSV-1.

PRODROME: An early warning symptom of illness, prodrome for a genital herpes outbreak often involves an aching, burning, itching, or tingling sensation in the genital area, buttocks, or legs.

PRODRUG: A medication that must undergo chemical conversion in the body in order to change to its active form.

RECURRENCE: The presence of lesions caused by reactivation of HSV ("outbreak").

STD: Sexually transmitted disease. See STI, sexually transmitted infections.

STI: Sexually transmitted infection; any infection that is acquired through sexual contact.

SACRAL GANGLION: The nerve root at the base of the spine that serves as the site of latency in genital herpes infections.

SEROLOGIC TEST: A test that identifies the antibodies in serum (a clear fluid that is a component of blood).

SEROSTATUS: A determination, based on serology, of whether a person has antibodies to any particular microbe—for example, HSV-1 or HSV-2.

STEROIDS: A group of drugs, including corticosteroids and anabolic steroids, that affect metabolism.

SYMPTOMATIC REACTIVATION: The presence of lesions or any other symptoms caused by reactivation of HSV; a "recurrence."

SYSTEMIC SYMPTOMS: Fever, headache, fatigue, or other symptoms of illness affecting the whole body, as distinguished from the surface lesions seen in a herpes recurrence.

TRANSMISSION: The spread of herpes from one person to another.

TRIGGER (FACTOR): Any biologic or behavioral event that influences latent HSV to reactivate.

TRUE PRIMARY EPISODE: A person's first infection with either type of HSV: a primary first episode. See "first episode."

VIRAL REPLICATION: The process by which a virus makes more copies of itself.

FURTHER READING

OVERVIEW OF GENITAL HERPES

Benedetti, J., Corey, L., Ashley, R. "Recurrence Rates in Genital Herpes after Symptomatic First-Episode Infections." *Annals of Internal Medicine* 1994; 12: 847-54.

Benedetti, J.K., Zeh, J., Corey, L. "Clinical reactivation of genital herpes simplex virus infection decreases in frequency over time." *Annals of Internal Medicine* 1999; 131(1): 14-20.

Engelberg, R., Carrell, D., Krantz, E., Corey, L., Wald, A. "Natural history of genital herpes simplex virus type 1 infection." *Sexually Transmitted Diseases* 2003 Feb; 30(2): 174-7.

Kerkering, K., Gardella, C., Selke, S., Krantz, E., Corey, L., Wald, A. "Isolation of Herpes Simplex Virus From the Genital Tract During Symptomatic Recurrence on the Buttocks." *Obstetrics and Gynecology* 2006; 108: 974.

Langenberg, A., Corey, L., Ashley, R., Leong, W.P., Straus, S. "A Prospective Study of New Infections with Herpes Simplex Virus Type 1 and Type 2." *New England Journal of Medicine* 1999; 341(19): 1432-1438.

Schillinger, J., Fujie, X. Sternberg, M., et al. "National Seroprevalence and Trends in Herpes Simplex Virus Type 1 in the United States. 1976-1994." *Sexually Transmitted Diseases* 2004; 31: 753-760.

Wald, A., Corey, L., Cone, R., Hobson, A., Davis, G., Zeh, J. "Frequent Genital Herpes Simplex Virus 2 Shedding in Immunocompetent Women: Effect of Acyclovir Treatment." *Journal of Clinical Investigation* 1997; 99(5): 1092-7.

Wald, A., Zeh, J., Selke, S. "Reactivation of genital herpes simplex virus type 2 infection in asymptomatic HSV-2 seropositive persons." *New England Journal of Medicine* 2000; 342: 844-850.

Wald, A., Zeh, J., Selke, S., Ashley, R., Corey, L. "Virologic Characteristics of Subclinical and Symptomatic Genital Herpes Infection." *New England Journal of Medicine* 1995; 333: 770-5.

Wald, A., Zeh, J., Selke, S., Warren, T., Ryncarz, AJ., Ashley, R., Krieger, JN., Corey, L. "Reactivation of genital herpes simplex virus type 2 infection in asymptomatic seropositive persons." *New England Journal of Medicine* 2000 Mar 23; 342(12): 844-50.

Xu, F., Sternberg, M., Kottiri, B., McQuillan, G., et al. "Trends in Herpes Simplex Virus Type 1 and Type 2 Seroprevalence in the United States." *Journal of the American Medical Association* 2006; 296: 964-972.

Zhu, J., Koelle, DM., Cao, J., Vazquez, J., Huang, ML., Hladik, F., Wald, A., Corey L. "Virus-specific CD8+ T cells accumulate near sensory nerve endings in genital skin during subclinical HSV-2 reactivation." *Journal of Experimental Medicine* 2007 Mar 19; 204(3): 595-603.

TRANSMISSION AND PREVENTION

Casper, C., Wald, A. "Condom use and the Prevention of Genital Herpes Acquisition." *Herpes* 2002; 9(1): 10-14.

Corey, L., Langenberg, A. G., Ashley, R., et al. "Recombinant glycoprotein vaccine for the prevention of genital HSV-2 infection: two randomized controlled trials." *Journal of the American Medical Association* 1999; 282(4): 331-40.

Corey, L., Wald, A., Celum, CL., Quinn, TC. "The effects of herpes simplex virus-2 on HIV-1 acquisition and transmission: a review of two overlapping epidemics." *Journal of Acquired Immune Deficiency Syndromes* 2004 Apr 15; 35(5): 435-45. Review.

Corey, L., Wald, A., Patel, R., Sacks SL., Tyring, SK., Warren, T., Douglas, JM. Jr., Paavonen, J., Morrow, RA., Beutner, KR., Stratchounsky, LS., Mertz, G., Keene, ON., Watson, HA., Tait, D., Vargas-Cortes, M. for the Valacyclovir HSV Transmission Study Group. "Once-daily valacyclovir to reduce the risk of transmission of genital herpes." *New England Journal of Medicine* 2004 Jan 1; 350(1): 11-20.

Drake, AL., John-Stewart, GC., Wald, A., Mbori-Ngacha, DA., Bosire, R., Wamalwa, DC., Lohman-Payne, BL., Ashley-Morrow, R., Corey, L., Farquhar, C. "Herpes simplex virus type 2 and risk of intrapartum human immunodeficiency virus transmission." *Obstetrics & Gynecology*. 2007 Feb; 109 (2 Pt 1): 403-9. Erratum in: *Obstetrics & Gynecology* 2007 Apr; 109(4): 1002-3.

Gottlieb, S., Douglas, J., Foster, M., et al. "Incidence of Herpes Simplex Virus Type 2 Infection in 5 Sexually Transmitted Disease (STD) Clinics and the Effect of HIV/STD Risk-reduction Counseling." *Journal of Infectious Diseases* 2004; 190: 1059-1067.

Kim, HN., Meier, A., Huang, ML., Kuntz, S., Selke, S., Celum, C., Corey, L., Wald, A. "Oral herpes simplex virus type 2 reactivation in HIV-positive and -negative men." *Journal of Infectious Diseases* 2006 Aug 15; 194(4): 420-7. Epub 2006 Jul 12.

Mertz, G., Benedetti, J., Ashley, R., Selke, S., Corey, L. "Risk Factors for the Sexual Transmission of Genital Herpes." *Annals of Internal Medicine* 1992; 116: 197-202.

Wald, A., Krantz, E., Selke, S., Lairson, E., Morrow, RA., Zeh, J. "Knowledge of partners' genital herpes protects against herpes simplex virus type 2 acquisition." *Journal of Infectious Diseases* 2006 Jul 1; 194(1): 42-52. Epub 2006 May 24.

Wald, A., Langenberg, A., et al. "Effect of Condoms on Reducing the Transmission of Herpes Simplex Virus Type 2 from Men to Women." *Journal of the American Medical Association* 2001; 285: 3100-3106.

Wald, A., Langenberg, AG., Krantz, E., Douglas, Jr., JM, Handsfield, HH., DiCarlo, RP., Adimora, AA., Izu, AE., Morrow, RA., Corey, L. "The relationship between condom use and herpes simplex virus acquisition." *Annals of Internal Medicine* 2005 Nov 15; 143(10): 707-13. Summary for patients in: *Annals of Internal Medicine* 2005 Nov 15; 143(10): I40.

Wald, A., Zeh, J., Barnum, G., Davis, G., Corey, L. "Suppression of Subclinical Shedding of Herpes Simplex Virus Type 2 with Acyclovir." *Annals of Internal Medicine* 1996; 124: 8-15.

TREATMENT OPTIONS

Aoki F.Y., Tyring S., Diaz-Mitoma F., Gross G., Gao J., Hamed K. "Single-day, patient-initiated famciclovir therapy for recurrent genital herpes: a randomized, double-blind, placebo-controlled trial." *Clinical Infectious Diseases* 2006; 42(1): 8-13.

Bryson, Y., Dillon, M., Lovett, M., Acuna, G., Taylor, S., Cherry, J., Johnson, L., Wiesmeier, E., Growdon, W., Creagh-Kirk, T., Keeney, R. "Treatment of First Episodes of Genital Herpes Simplex Virus Infection with Oral Acyclovir: A Randomized Double-Blind Controlled Trial in Normal Subjects." *New England Journal of Medicine* Apr 1983; 308: 916-21.

Centers for Disease Control and Prevention. "Recommendations and

Reports." *MMWR* 2006; Vol. 55/RR-11: 16-23.

Corey, L., Wald, A., Patel, R., et al. "Once-daily Valacyclovir to Reduce the Risk of Transmission of Genital Herpes." *New England Journal of Medicine* 2004; 350: 11-20.

Fife, K., Crumpacker, C., Mertz, G., Hill, E., Boone, G., and the Acyclovir Study Group. "Recurrence and Resistance Patterns of Herpes Simplex Virus Following Cessation of Greater than or Equal to Six Years of Chronic Suppression with Acyclovir." *Journal of Infectious Diseases* 1994; 169: 1338-41.

Goldberg, L., Kaufman, R., Kurtz, T., Conant, M., Eron, L., Batenhorst, R., Boone, G. and the Acyclovir Study Group. "Long-Term Suppression of Recurrent Genital Herpes with Acyclovir: A 5-Year Benchmark." *Archives of Dermatology* 1993; 129: 582-7.

Gupta, R., Wald, A., Krantz, E., Selke, S., Warren, T., Vargas-Cortes, M., Miller, G., Corey, L. "Valacyclovir and acyclovir for suppression of shedding of herpes simplex virus in the genital tract." *Journal of Infectious Diseases* 2004 Oct 15; 190(8): 1374-81. Epub 2004 Sep 20.

Kaplowitz, L., Baker, D., Gelb, L., Blythe, J., Hale, R., Frost, P., Crumpacker, C., Rabinovich, S., Peacock, J., Herndon, J., Davis, G., and the Acyclovir Study Group. "Prolonged Continuous Acyclovir Treatment of Normal Adults with Frequently Recurring Genital Herpes Simplex Virus Infection." *Journal of the American Medical Association* 1991; 256(6): 747-51.

Kost, R., Hill, E., Tigges, M., Straus, S. "Brief Report: Recurrent Acyclovir-Resistant Genital Herpes in an Immunocompetent Patient." *New England Journal of Medicine* 1993; 329(24): 1777-82.

Mark, KE., Corey, L., Meng, TC., Magaret, AS., Huang ML., Selke, S., Slade, HB., Tyring, SK., Warren, T., Sacks, SL., Leone, P., Bergland, VA., Wald, A. "Topical resiquimod 0.01% gel decreases herpes simplex virus type 2 genital shedding: a randomized, controlled trial." *Journal of Infectious Diseases* 2007 May 1; 195(9): 1324-31.

Mertz, G., Loveless, M., Levin, M., Kraus, S., Fowler, S., Goade, D., Tyring, S. "Oral Famciclovir for Suppression of Recurrent Genital Herpes Simplex Virus Infection in Women." *Archives of Internal Medicine* 1997; 157: 343.

Patel, R., Tyring, S., Strand, A., Price M.J., Grant, D.M. "Impact of suppressive antiviral therapy on the health-related quality of life of patients with recurrent genital herpes infection." *Sexually Transmitted Infections* 1999; 75: 398-402.

Safrin, S., Crumpacker, C., Chatis, P., Davis, R., Hafner, R., Rush, J., Kessler, H., Landry, B., Mills, J., and other members of the AIDS Clinical Trials Group. "A Controlled Trial Comparing Foscarnet with Vidarabine for Acyclovir-Resistant Mucocutaneous Herpes Simplex in the Acquired Immunodeficiency Syndrome." *New England Journal of Medicine* 1991; 325(8): 551-5.

Wald, A., Carrell, D., Remington, M., Kexel, E., Zeh, J., Corey, L. "Two-day regimen of acyclovir for treatment of recurrent genital herpes simplex virus type 2 infection." *Clinical Infectious Diseases* 2002 Apr 1; 34(7): 944-8. Epub 2002 Feb 20.

Wald, A., Selke, S., Warren, T., Aoki, F.Y., Sacks, S., Diaz-Mitoma, F., Corey, L. "Comparative efficacy of famciclovir and valacyclovir for suppression of recurrent genital herpes and viral shedding." *Sexually Transmitted Diseases* 2006 Sep; 33(9): 529-33.

Whitley, R., Gnann, J. "Acyclovir: A Decade Later." *New England Journal of Medicine* 1992; 327: 782-9.

TAKING CONTROL—THE EMOTIONAL ISSUES

Aral, S., VanderPlate, C., Magder, L. "Recurrent Genital Herpes: What Helps Adjustment?" *Sexually Transmitted Diseases* 1988; 15(3): 164-6.

Brookes, J., Haywood, S., and Green, J. "Adjustment to the psychological and social sequelae of recurrent genital herpes simplex infection." *Genitourinary Medicine* 1993; 69: 384-7.

Carney, O., et al., "A prospective study of the psychological impact on patients with a first episode of genital herpes." *Genitourinary Medicine* 1994; 70: 40-45.

Catotti, D., Clarke, P., Catoe, K. "Herpes Revisited: Still a Cause of Concern." *Sexually Transmitted Diseases* 1993; 20(2): 77-80.

Mindel, A., "Psychological and psychosexual implications of herpes simplex virus infections." *Scandinavian Journal of Infectious Diseases Supplement* 1996; 100: 27-32.

Swanson, J., Dibble, S., Chenitz, W. "Clinical features and psychosocial factors in young adults with genital herpes." *Journal of Nursing Scholarship* 1995; 27: 16-22.

COMPLEMENTARY AND ALTERNATIVE MEDICINE

Longo, D. "Psychosocial Treatment for Recurrent Genital Herpes." *Journal of Consulting and Clinical Psychology* 1988; 56(1). 61-66.

Perfect, M.M., Bourne, N., Ebel, C., & Rosenthal, S.L. "Use of Complementary and Alternative Medicine for the Treatment of Genital Herpes." *Herpes* 2005; 12(2): 38-41.

Rooney, J., Bryson, Y., Mannix, M., Dillon, M., Wohlenberg, C., Banks, S., Wallington, C., Notkins, A., Straus, S. "Prevention of

Ultraviolet-Light-Induced Herpes Labialis by Sunscreen." *Lancet* 1991; 338(8180): 1419-22.

HERPES AND PREGNANCY

Arvin, A., Hensleigh, P., Prober, C., Au, D., Yasukawa, L., Wittek, A., Palumbo, P., Paryani, S., Yeager, S. "Failure of Antepartum Maternal Cultures to Predict the Infant's Risk of Exposure to Herpes Simplex Virus at Delivery." *New England Journal of Medicine* 1986; 315(13): 796-800.

Brown, ZA., Gardella, C., Wald, A., Morrow, RA., Corey, L. "Genital herpes complicating pregnancy." *Obstetrics & Gynecology* 2005 Oct; 106(4):845-56. Review. Erratum in: *Obstetrics & Gynecology* 2006 Feb; 107(2 Pt 1): 428. *Obstetrics & Gynecology* 2007 Jan; 109(1): 207.

Brown, Z., Selke, M., Zeh, J., Kopelman, J., Maslow, A., Ashley, R., Watts, H., Berry, S., Herd, M., Corey, L. "The Acquisition of Herpes Simplex Virus during Pregnancy." *New England Journal of Medicine* 1997; 337(8): 509-15.

Brown, ZA., Wald, A., Morrow, RA., Selke, S., Zeh, J., Corey, L. "Effect of serologic status and cesarean delivery on transmission rates of herpes simplex virus from mother to infant." *Journal of American Medical Association* 2003 Jan 8; 289(2): 203-9.

Chen, KT., Segu, M., Lumey, LH., Kuhn, L., Carter, RJ., Bulterys, M., Abrams, EJ., New York City Perinatal AIDS Collaborative Transmission Study (PACTS) Group. "Genital herpes simplex virus infection and perinatal transmission of human immunodeficiency virus." *Obstetric & Gynecology* 2005 Dec; 106(6): 1341-8.

Cone, R., Hobson, A., Brown, Z., Ashley, R., Berry, S., Winter, C., Corey, L. "Frequent Detection of Genital Herpes Simplex Virus DNA by Polymerase Chain Reaction among Pregnant Women." *Journal of the*

American Medical Association 1994; 272 (10): 792-6.

Gardella, C., Brown, Z., et al. "Poor Correlation Between Genital Lesions and Detection of Herpes Simplex Virus in Women in Labor." *Obstetrics & Gynecology* 2005; 106: 268-274

Gardella, C., Brown, Z., Wald, A., Selke, S., Zeh, J., Morrow, RA., Corey, L. "Risk factors for herpes simplex virus transmission to pregnant women: a couples study." *American Journal of Obstetrics & Gynecology* 2005 Dec; 193(6): 1891-9.

Handsfield, H., Waldo A., Brown Z., Corey L., Drucker J., Ebel C., Leone P., Stanberry L., Whitley R. "Neonatal Herpes Should Be a Reportable Disease." *Sexually Transmitted Diseases* Sept. 2005; 32(9): 521-525.

Kulhanjian, J., Soroush, V., Au, D., Bronzan, R., Yasukawa, L., Weylman, L., Arvin, A., Prober, C. "Identification of Women at Unsuspected Risk of Primary Infection with Herpes Simplex Virus Type 2 during Pregnancy." *New England Journal of Medicine* 1992; 326(14): 916-20.

Randolph, A., Washington, E., Prober, C. "Cesarean Delivery for Women Presenting with Genital Herpes Lesions: Efficacy, Risks, and Costs." *Journal of the American Medical Association* 1993; 270(1): 77.

Scott, L., Sanchez, P., Jackson, G., Zeray, F., Wendel, G. "Acyclovir Suppression to Prevent Cesarean Delivery after First-Episode Genital Herpes." *Obstetrics & Gynecology* 1996; 87(1): 69-73.

Whitley, R., Arvin, A., Prober, C., Corey, L., Burchett, S., Plotkin, S., Staff, S., Jacobs, R., Powell, D., Nahmias, A., Sumaya, C., Edwards, K., Alford, C., Caddell, G., Soong, S., and the National Institute of Allergy and Infectious Diseases Collaborative Antiviral Study Group.

"Predictors of Morbidity and Mortality in Neonates with Herpes Simplex Virus Infections." *New England Journal of Medicine* 1991; 324(7): 450-4.

THE BROADER SPECTRUM OF HSV INFECTION

Belongia, E., Goodman, J., Holland, E., Andres, C., Homann, S., Mahanti, R., Mizener, M., Erice, A., Osterhold, M. "An Outbreak of Herpes Gladiatorum at a High-School Wrestling Camp." *New England Journal of Medicine* 1991; 325(13): 906-10.

Bergstrom, T., Vahlne, A., Alestig, K., Jeansson, S., Forsgren, M., Lycke, E. "Primary and Recurrent Herpes Simplex Virus Type 2-Induced Meningitis." *Journal of Infectious Diseases* 1990; 162: 327.

Cherpes, TL., Meyn, LA., Hillier, SL. "Cunnilingus and vaginal intercourse are risk factors for herpes simplex virus type 1 acquisition in women." *Sexually Transmitted Diseases* 2005 Feb; 32(2): 84-9.

Cherpes, TL., Meyn, LA., Krohn, MA., Lurie, JG., Hillier, SL. "Association between acquisition of herpes simplex virus type 2 in women and bacterial vaginosis." *Clinical Infectious Diseases* 2003 Aug 1; 37(3): 319-25. Epub 2003 July 15.

Gill, J., Arlette, J., Buchan, K. "Herpes Simplex Virus Infection of the Hand." *American Journal of Medicine* 1988; 84: 89-91.

Klotz, R. "Herpetic Whitlow: An Occupational Hazard." *Journal of the American Association of Nurse Anesthetists* 1990; 58(1): 8-13.

DIAGNOSIS

Ashley, R. "Inability of Enzyme Immunoassay to Discriminate between Infections with Herpes Simplex Virus Types 1 and 2." *Annals of Internal Medicine* 1991; 115: 520.

Ashley, R.L., Wald, A., "Genital herpes: review of the epidemic and potential use of type-specific serology." *Clinical Microbiology Reviews* 1999; 12(1): 1-8.

Fairley, I., Monteiro, E. F. "Patient attitudes to type-specific serologic tests in the diagnosis of genital herpes." *Genitourin Medicine* 1997; 73: 259-262.

Miyai, T., Turner, KR., Kent, CK., Klausner, J. "The psychosocial impact of testing individuals with no history of genital herpes for herpes simplex virus type 2." *Sexually Transmitted Diseases* 2004 Sep; 31(9): 517-21.

Richards, J., Scholes, D., Caka, S., Drolette, L., Magaret, AM., Yarbro, P., Lafferty, W., Crosby, R., Diclemente, R., Wald, A. "HSV 2 Serologic Testing in an HMO Population: Uptake and Psychosocial Sequelae." *Sexually Transmitted Diseases* 2007 Apr 26.

Rosenthal, SL., Zimet, GD., Leichliter, JS., Stanberry, LR., Fife, KH., Tu, W., Bernstein, DI. "The psychosocial impact of serological diagnosis of asymptomatic herpes simplex virus type 2 infection." *Sexually Transmitted Infections* 2006 Apr; 82(2): 154-7; discussion 157 8.

OTHER STIS

Dunne, E., Unger, E., Sternberg, M., McQuillan, G., Swan, D., Patel, S., Markowitz, L. "Prevalence of HPV Infection Among Females in the United States." *Journal of the American Medical Association* 2007; 297(8): 813-819.

Weinstock, H., Berman, S., Cates Jr., W. "Sexually Transmitted Diseases Among American Youth: Incidence and Prevalence Estimates, 2000." *Perspectives on Sexual and Reproductive Health* 2004; 36: 7-10.

Weller, S., Stanberry, L., "Estimating the Population Prevalence of HPV." *Journal of the American Medical Association* 2007; 297(8): 876-878.

INDEX

Garlic, 107. *See also* alternative therapy, herbal remedies, treatment (alternative).

Genital herpes, 1-3, 5-6, 9-10, 12-13, 15-20, 24, 26-29, 33-5, 55-59, 62, 65, 67-79, 81, 83-86, 88-90, 94-95, 98, 101-108, 111, 120, 126-127, 132, 137-139, 141, 146, 151-159, 162-163, 165-166, 168, 170, 172, 231. *See also* complications, diagnosis, emotional issues, first episode, HSV (herpes simplex virus), HSV-1, HSV-2, recurrent genital herpes, symptoms, transmission, treatment, triggers

long-term patterns, 8
prevalence, 12-13, 68
symptoms, 9, 44-46, 70-71

Genital warts/HPV (human papillomavirus), 204. *See also* sexually transmitted infections.

GlaxoSmithKline (GSK), 83, 191-193, 197, 205, 224

Gonorrhea, 2, 162, 202-203, 207-208. *See also* sexually transmitted infections.

Health insurance coverage, 79, 98, 217-220

Healthcare provider, 26-27, 29, 36, 43, 45, 71-75, 77, 80, 86, 91, 115-116, 154-155, 162-163, 174-175, 179, 182-183, 185, 207, 209

discussing emotional issues, 73-75, 77, 98, 116
importance of, 73

pregnancy, 154-155, 162-163

Healthy lifestyle, 113. *See also* immune system, treatments.

Helper, The (ASHA newsletter), 199

Hepatitis, *See* virus/viruses.

Hepatitis B, 194, 205, 207. *See also* sexually transmitted infections.

Herbal remedies, 105, 107, 109. *See also* alternative therapy, treatment (alternative).

HerpeSelect™ 1 & 2 ELISA, 179-180

HerpeSelect™ 1 & 2 Immunoblot, 179

Herpes encephalitis, 160, 168-169, 175, 231. *See also* encephalitis (herpes).

Herpes gladiatorum (wrestler's herpes), 58, 231

Herpes simplex virus (HSV). *See* HSV.

Herpetic whitlow, 166-167, 172, 231. *See also* complications.

Herpes Testing Toolkit, 179, 182

Herpesvirus, 6-8, 34, 78, 104, 112, 177, 186, 197, 208, 232. *See also* virus/viruses.

HIV/AIDS, 5, 15, 94-95, 123, 139, 162, 169-170, 172, 177, 184, 198, 205-209, 212. *See also* sexually transmitted infections.

behavioral link, 139-140
criminal law, 212-213
herpes treatment, 94
link to HSV, STIs, 139-140, 184
prevention, 150, 198, 207-209

Hotlines

National Herpes Hotline, 55, 80,

127, 173, 211, 221
STI Resource Center Hotline, 183,
206, 222
HPV, 204-205. *See also* genital warts.
HSV (herpes simplex virus), 3, 5, 8-13,
20, 23, 25-27, 29-31, 34-37, 40,
43-45, 48, 52-53, 55-56, 58, 60-
65, 68-71, 77, 82-85, 87-89, 90-
96, 101-104, 106-109, 112, 115,
128, 132-135, 139-140, 146, 151-
160, 165, 167-173, 231. *See also*
diagnosis, HSV-1, HSV-2, sexually
transmitted infections, transmission, treatment, virus/viruses.
legal issues, 211-217
prevalence of, 12, 15, 93, 198, 202-
204
symptoms, 25-28, 36-46
testing, 179, 184
types, 6-8, 165
HSV-1, 231
blood test, 1, 15-19, 49-50, 67, 72,
128, 144, 177, 183, 186
differences from HSV-2, 176
frequency of recurrence, 46-50,112,
145
prevalence of, 12-13, 140, 145
sites of preference, 10, 45
sunlight (ultraviolet light), 51
superinfection, 28
symptoms, 8-9, 13, 25-26
transmission, 9-10, 13, 145, 158
triggers, 50-52
type-specific tests, 29, 76, 176

HSV-2, 231
blood test, 1, 15-19, 49-50, 67, 72,
128, 144, 177, 183, 186
differences from HSV-1, 144, 176
frequency of recurrence, 46-50, 145
history vs. no history, 16
prevalence of, 12-13, 145, 177
sites of preference, 8, 45
symptoms, 8-9, 13, 25-26
transmission, 9-10, 113, 145
triggers, 50-52
type-specific test, 29, 76, 176-180
Human Herpesvirus Type 6 (HHV-6),
6. *See also* herpesviruses.
Human Herpesvirus Type 7 (HHV-7),
6. *See also* herpesviruses.
Human Herpesvirus Type 8 (HHV-8),
6. *See also* herpesviruses.
Human papillomavirus (HPV). *See*
HPV.
Humoral immune response, 24
Hydrocortisone, 30, 104
Immune modulators, 95
Immune system, 6-8, 10, 13, 24-27, 34,
60, 84-85, 89, 92-93, 1010, 136,
154, 159, 168, 190, 193, 195,
197, 204, 206
cellular immune response, 24, 190,
194
compromised, 169, 172
HIV/AIDS, 208
humoral immune response, 24
immune response, 13, 24-25, 59, 85,
92, 95, 157, 166, 177, 190-191,
194-197

INDEX

182, 230
accuracy, 174-175
cell culture, 174-175, 230
cost, 175
first episodes, 174-175
pregnancy, 160
sensitivity, 174-175
specificity, 174-175
Viral infection, 5, 7, 74, 89, 95, 103, 126, 201, 205. *See also* virus/viruses
Viral replication, 7, 85, 95, 103, 234
Viral shedding. *See* reactivation, subclinical shedding, transmission.
Viral type, 45, 53, 70, 176-177, 193
Virus/viruses, 6-8
  cytomegalovirus, 6
  Epstein-Barr virus (mononucleosis), 6
  herpes simplex virus (HSV), 3, 5, 8, 16, 23, 34, 55, 63, 65, 73, 126, 174, 189
  hepatitis, 5, 190, 194, 205
  herpesvirus, 6-8, 34, 78, 104, 112, 177, 186, 197, 208
  human papillomavirus (HPV), 187, 204-205, 213
  varicella zoster virus (shingles, chicken pox), 6, 8, 43, 197, 208, 232
Vitamins/vitamin supplements, 107, 108. *See also* alternative therapy, nutrition.
Western blot, 179, 180. *See also* diagnosis/diagnostic test.
Wrestler's herpes, 58-59, 231. *See also* herpes gladiatorum.

Xylocaine, 104
Zinc, 107
Zovirax®, 82, 102. *See also* acyclovir.

259

MANAGING HERPES